Carole

Focus on Corona

Focus on Coronary Care

Joy McCulloch
RGN, BSc *Social Sciences/Nursing Studies, DN,*
Sister on CCU

Ann Townsend
SRN, *Senior Sister on CCU*

David O. Williams
FRCP (Lond.) FRCP (Edin.) *Consultant Cardiologist*

William Heinemann Medical Books
London

First published 1985 by William Heinemann Medical Books Ltd
23 Bedford Square, London WC1B 3HH

ISBN: 0–433–32630–1

Typeset by Inforum Ltd, Portsmouth
Printed in Great Britain at The Pitman Press, Bath

Contents

Foreword

The intensive care of those suspected of having sustained a myocardial infarction is now more than 20 years old, but the knowledge and skills of those working in this field have been constantly undergoing change as new methods of diagnosis and treatment have been developed. From the inception of coronary care units, nurses have played a key role and exceptional responsibilities have developed onto them because of the special and unusual situation that arises in acute myocardial infarction; the patient may be fully alert yet in danger of sudden but unpredictable death. This means that the nurse (and the junior medical staff) must be ready to act promptly and effectively at a moment's notice and without recourse to more experienced individuals. It is thus vital that those responsible for the care of patients with myocardial infarction should understand the nature of the disorder, be able to recognise and treat its complications, and be familiar with the many new drugs now available as well as the specialised techniques such as pacemaking and cardioversion. In an increasing number of units, nurses must be able to cope with haemodynamic monitoring and the intra-aortic balloon pump. In all they must have as a primary concern the psychological problems that arise both in the patient and in those close to him or her.

This book provides a succinct and practical guide to staff involved in the care of those acutely ill with cardiac disorders and should prove particularly useful to those who wish to make themselves familiar with current ideas on management in this vitally important area of medicine.

3 December 1984 — Professor D.G. JULIAN
British Heart Foundation Professor of Cardiology
Freeman Hospital
Newcastle-upon-Tyne

Acknowledgements

The people we would like to acknowledge are:
  Mrs L. Walton, Nursing Officer, for her contribution of Chapter 14.
  Yvonne Townsend for her help with graphics.
  Eleanor Allman, Julie and all other secretarial help.
  Jeffrey Pearson for his photographic assistance.
  Husbands, wives and friends for their support and encouragement.

1

History and Development of Coronary Care Units

In the Western world about fifty per cent of all deaths are due to cardiovascular disease. Of these deaths, half are attributed to ischaemic heart disease. This is particularly common in males in the mid-fifty age group, although it is now seen more frequently in younger people. Many patients who suffer from a heart attack die within the first few hours, ventricular fibrillation being the most common cause of sudden death. The first physician to diagnose myocardial infarction in the United Kingdom was McNee of Glasgow in 1925. Since then a great deal has been discovered about the physiology and pathology of myocardial infarction and it is now accepted that prompt action and new methods of treatment will improve mortality rates.

It is over 200 years since Heberden described that patients with angina pectoris may die suddenly. Jenner, the discoverer of smallpox vaccine, associated angina pectoris with coronary artery disease in the early nineteenth century. Experimental work continued throughout the nineteenth and the first half of the twentieth century, but it was not until 1947 that a human heart was defibrillated. In 1947 Beck *et al.* successfully applied cardiac massage and electrical defibrillation through a thoracotomy to a young 14-year-old boy, who had developed ventricular fibrillation following chest surgery. As a result of this work, surgeons were trained in the technique of open chest defibrillation. Nine years later in 1956, Beck *et al.* applied the same techniques to a 65-year-old physician who developed ventricular fibrillation following myocardial infaction. Reagan *et al.* also used open chest defribrillation to successfully resuscitate a patient who developed an arrhythmia while having an electrocardiogram recorded. In 1956 Zoll and his colleagues demonstrated that ventricular fibrillation could be abolished by defibrillation externally to the chest wall. Work continued in this field and in 1960 Kouwenhoven *et al.* showed that the heart could be massaged without thoracotomy. Combined with mouth to mouth respiration, this closed massage would maintain an oxygenated blood supply to vital organs until external defibrillation could be applied.

Resuscitation from ventricular fibrillation was becoming a reality and in 1961 Julian suggested that 'all medical, nursing and auxiliary staff should be trained in the techniques of closed chest massage and mouth to mouth breathing' (Julian, 1961). He also suggested that 'patients known to be at risk should have their cardiac rhythm constantly monitored'. In 1962 Coronary Care Units (CCUs) were established — Julian opening a unit in Sydney, Day in Kansas City, Brown in Toronto and Meltzer in Philadelphia. In the United Kingdom, an area designated for the management of the patient with acute myocardial infarction was opened by Shillingford in 1963 at the Hammersmith Hospital. The first unit to routinely receive patients with infarction was opened by Julian and Oliver in Edinburgh in 1968.

The original concept of the CCU was the resuscitation of patients with ventricular fibrillation following myocardial infarction, in a segregated environment under the care of both medical and nursing staff trained to use specialised equipment. Attention was then directed to the prevention of arrhythmias. The World Health Organisation also recognised the need for research and treatment in coronary care and a booklet with guidelines in setting up CCUs and training of staff was published. Because of the high death rate outside hospital, Pantridge in Belfast extended the concept of coronary care into the community by equipping and staffing ambulances in 1966. This introduced the concept of mobile coronary care units (MCCUs).

Since those early days, the role of the CCU has expanded as a result of new drugs, new techniques and the expertise of both medical and nursing staff. This is particularly applicable to the larger centres of cardiology where patients other than those suffering myocardial infarction are admitted for treatment (see Chapter 13).

Other patients who may be admitted to the CCU include the unstable angina pectoris group who are susceptible to sudden death due to infarction and ventricular dysrhythmia. Some of these may require the aid of the intra aortic balloon pump to help them over the critical part of their illness. Diagnostic cardiac catheterisation and coronary angiography can then take place, allowing decisions to be made about whether the patient should undergo a coronary artery bypass graft. Other patients in cardiogenic shock due to mechanical causes may also benefit from intra aortic balloon counterpulsation techniques, including those with ventricular septal defect and papillary muscle dysfunction following myocardial infarction (see Chapter 11). Another recent advance of coronary care is the management of patients with cardiac failure which may be due either to acute or chronic heart disease. Early work by Swan and Ganz has led to the use of haemodynamic monitoring in association with drug therapy in the treatment of these patients (see Chapter 12).

Although CCUs have a relatively short history, they have made an impression, not only on the management of patients with a diagnosis of myocardial infarction, but also in the treatment of those with arrhythmias and severe heart failure. Cost and efficiency are always under discussion in CCUs as in all intensive care units, but CCUs will remain with us in some form as an accepted part of the hospital service. Therefore, it is important that the training of both medical and nursing staff is of the highest standard. This book is aimed at these personnel.

References and further reading

Beck C.S., Pritchard W.H., Feil H.S. (1947). Ventricular fibrillation of long duration abolished by electric shock. *Journal of the American Medical Association;* **135**:985–986.

Beck C.S., Weckesser E.C., Barry F.M. (1956). Fatal heart attack and successful defibrillation; new concepts of the coronary artery disease. *Journal of the American Medical Association;* **161**:434–436.

Julian D.G. (1961). Treatment of cardiac arrest in acute myocardial ischaemia and infarction. *Lancet;* **II**:840–844.

Kouwenhoven W.B., Jude J.R., Knickerbocker G.G. (1960). Closed chest massage. *Journal of the American Medical Association;* **173**:1064–1067.

Pantridge J.F. Geddes J.S. (1967). A mobile intensive care unit in the management of myocardial infarction. *Lancet;* **II**:271–273.

Reagan L.B., Young K.R., Nicholson J.W. (1956). Ventricular fibrillation in a patient with probable acute coronary occlusion. *Surgery;* **39**:482–486.

Zoll P.M., Linethal A.J., Gibson W., Paul M.H., Norman C.R. (1956). Termination of ventricular fibrillation in man by externally applied electric countershock. *New England Journal of Medicine;* **254**:727–732.

2

The Basics of Cardiac Anatomy and Physiology

ANATOMY

The heart is an organ of specialised muscle. Its primary function is to contract and relax, pumping blood around the body and perfusing all vital organs with oxygenated blood.

The heart is often described as a hollow, cone-shaped organ with muscular walls. It is said to be approximately the size of the owner's fist and to weigh about 270 g.

The apex of the heart lies downwards and to the left; the base lies above and medially (Fig. 2.1). The heart is situated between the lungs in the mediastinum. Its right side is in an anterior position under the sternum; the left side lies posteriorly and inferiorly. However, the position of the heart may alter with respiration due to its close proximity to the diaphragm.

Layers of the Heart's Wall

The three main structures which make up the heart wall are the:

1. pericardium.
2. myocardium.
3. endocardium (Fig. 2.2).

The pericardium is composed of two sacs: the tough outer fibrous

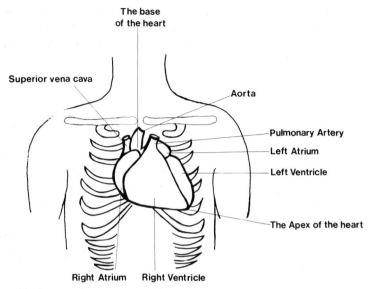

Fig. 2.1   *The position of the heart in the body.*

pericardium and the double inner layer of serous pericardium. The pericardial cavity is the name given to the potential space between the two layers of serous pericardium.

The myocardium is made up of a special kind of tissue known as cardiac muscle. This layer of involuntary muscle is thin at the base of the heart and thicker towards the apex. It is continuous over the heart except at the junction between the upper and lower chambers, where rings of fibrous tissue exist.

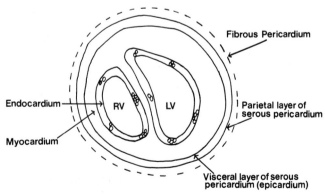

Fig. 2.2   *The layers of the heart's wall.*

The endocardium is the inner layer of the heart. It is lined with endothelial cells and is continuous with the tunica intima of the blood vessels. The myocardium and endocardium are bound together by connective tissue.

The Chambers of the Heart

The heart is divided into four chambers (Fig. 2.3): the right and left atria above and the right and left ventricles below.

The atria function mainly as collecting chambers and their contraction contributes only one-sixth to ventricular filling. The ventricles are the main pumping chambers of the heart. Disturbance of their function due to disease or arrhythmias has a more profound effect on cardiac output than atrial disturbances. The right ventricle is crescent-shaped on cross section. Its main muscles are the three papillary muscles and the moderator band. The walls of the left ventricle are approximately four times as thick as those of the right ventricle and it is circular in cross section. The

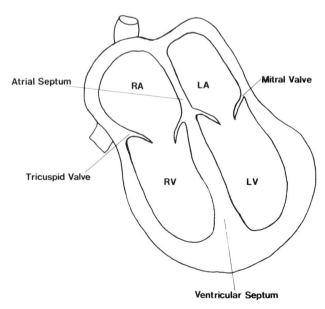

Fig. 2.3 The chambers of the heart.

main muscle projections of its walls are the two papillary muscles.

The chambers on the right side of the heart are separated from those on the left side by the septum, a division composed of muscle and lined with endocardium. In normal health, no blood should pass through the septum between the right and left sides of the heart.

The Atrioventricular Valves

The upper and lower chambers of each side of the heart are separated from each other by valves which are made up of folds of endocardium and fibrous tissue. The tricuspid valve which lies between the right atrium and right ventricle has three main cusps; the mitral valve which lies between the left atrium and left ventricle has two main cusps.

Attached to the lower outer edges of the main cusps of the atrioventricular valves are thin thread-like fibrous strands called chordae tendineae. The chordae tendineae are extensions of the papillary muscles of the ventricular walls. The atrioventricular (AV) valves open and close as a result of the pressure changes in the atria and ventricles. When the ventricular myocardium contracts, the papillary muscles tense. The valve cusps are prevented from being pushed back into the atria by the chordae tendineae. The valves ensure that the blood flows in the correct direction through the heart.

Outflow Valves

Valves are also present where the main blood vessels leave the ventricles. These are the pulmonary and aortic valves, which are termed semi-lunar valves.

Heart Sounds

The closure of the heart's valves is thought to be responsible for the first and second heart sounds. Both AV valves contribute to the first sound. It occurs at the onset of ventricular systole and is primarily due to the tensing of the valve cusps as ventricular pressure rises. The second heart sound is due to the closure of the aortic valve followed quickly by the closure of the pulmonary valve. The first and second heart sounds are responsible for the 'lub dub' often described as what is heard on auscultation of the normal heart.

Blood Flow Through the Heart (Fig. 2.4)

The superior and inferior vena cavae (SVC and IVC) are the largest veins of the body. They empty their blood into the right atrium (RA). The SVC and IVC open into the upper and lower aspects of the RA respectively. The RA also receives venous blood from the coronary sinus which drains the heart wall and opens onto the posterior surface of the RA just above the IVC. Other smaller veins from the heart wall also drain into the RA.

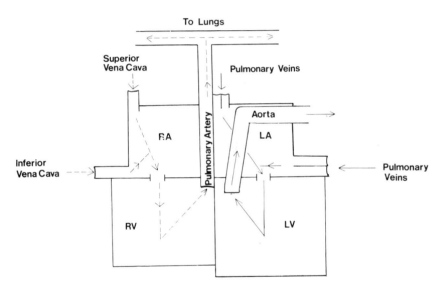

Fig. 2.4   A schematic representation of the blood flow through the heart.

Deoxygenated blood flows from the RA, through the tricuspid valve to the right ventricle (RV). Blood is ejected from here over the smooth walled pulmonary outflow tract, through the pulmonary valve and into the pulmonary artery. This is the only artery in the body to carry deoxygenated blood. This blood is transported to the lungs where carbon dioxide is excreted and oxygen is absorbed before it flows to the left atrium (LA) through the four pulmonary veins. Oxygenated blood flows from the LA through the mitral valve to the left ventricle (LV). High pressure builds up in the LV during systole, forcing the blood into the aorta and the systemic circulation.

The Special Conduction System of the Heart

Some parts of the cardiac muscle are composed of specialised cells which can produce and conduct the electrical impulses which result in cardiac contraction. In health, the impulses are produced at the sino-atrial node (SA node) which is situated in the RA at the top of the crista terminalis and close to the opening of the SVC (Fig. 2.5). Many cardiologists have investigated the possibility of the existence of specialised pathways of conduction in the atria — referred to as internodal tracts by some authors. The current feeling is that such tracts do not exist, although there are certain preferred pathways of atrial conduction. The only structure to pierce the fibrous tissue which separates the atria and ventricles is the specialised tissue of the bundle of His. The superior extremity of this is called the atrioventricular node (AV node). Together the AV node and the bundle of His are referred to as the AV junction. The bundle of His divides into the right and left bundle branches supplying the right and left ventricles respectively. The left bundle branch further divides into two fascicles, one passing superiorly and anteriorly through the LV, the other extending posteriorly and inferiorly. The fascicles of the right and left bundles further divide into many tiny branches called Purkinje fibres which carry the impulses into the ventricular myocardium (Fig. 2.5).

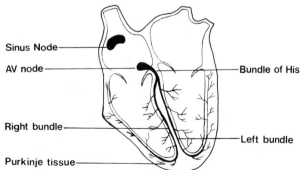

Fig. 2.5   The conduction system of the heart.

Normal electrical impulses produced at the SA node pass through the atrial myocardium before they enter the AV node and continue along the bundle of His. They travel down the right and left bundle branches and are then conducted into the ventricular myocardium, initiating ventricular contraction.

PHYSIOLOGY

The heart is composed of two main kinds of cells:

1. automatic, which produce the initial electrical stimulation for the myocardial cells and
2. myocardial, which provide the main pumping action of the heart.

The primary physiological properties of these cells are: automaticity, conduction and contraction.

Automaticity is the property by which certain areas of specialised heart muscle can initiate impulses. The cells in these areas may be called automatic or pacemaker cells. The pacemaker cells of the SA node initiate impulses at a rate of approximately 70 times a minute in a healthy, resting individual. However, should the SA node slow or stop, another area of automatic cells may take over as the pacemaker. Certain parts of the atria have this property of automaticity. The AV junctional area can produce and conduct impulses at a rate of 40–60 a minute. The ventricles may produce impulses at a rate of less than 40. These lower sites of impulse formation are called latent pacemakers. Sometimes a latent pacemaker will accelerate its rate of discharge and thus assume the role of pacemaker of the heart.

Conduction is a property of all heart cells. Both automatic and myocardial cells can conduct impulses. Conduction involves the passage of an impulse to an adjacent cell. The specialised tissue of the conduction system allows for the transmission of impulses in a rapid and organised manner.

Contraction is the main function of the myocardial cells; automatic cells have little of this property. Contraction is produced when the fibres of the cells shorten following electrical stimulation. Within physiological limits, the greater the diastolic volume, the greater the strength of contraction (Starling's law).

Electrophysiology: Action Potential of Myocardial Cells

The body is composed of electrolyte solutions in which electrical currents will flow. In resting myocardial cells, the inside is relatively negative in charge compared with the outside (Fig. 2.6). There is a potential difference in electricity across the cell membrane of approximately -90 millivolts (mV). These cells are called 'polarised' cells. If they are stimulated or injured, a change will take place in membrane permeability; an electrode placed across the cell membrane would then record a potential difference of $+20$mV. The change by which the inside of a cell becomes more positive in relation to the outside is called depolarisation. A depolarised cell is electrically negative on the outside compared with the neighbouring non-stimulated cells. A potential difference therefore exists and a current flows between all the cells until they have all been depolarised.

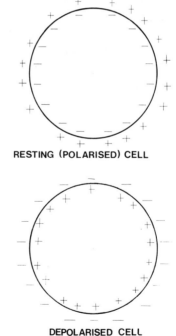

RESTING (POLARISED) CELL

DEPOLARISED CELL

Fig. 2.6 The electrical charges on a polarised and a depolarised myocardial cell.

Sodium and Potassium

The principal ions involved in the production of action potentials in the heart are potassium (K^+) and sodium (Na^+). There is a high concentration of K^+ within resting cells, whereas the extracellular concentration of K^+ is low. In contrast resting cells actively expel Na^+ by the sodium pump and thus the extracellular concentration of Na^+ is high. When the cell is stimulated, Na^+ ions enter the cell. As threshold potential (-60 mV) is reached, there is a further increase in permeability of the cell membrane to Na^+, another rush of Na^+ enters the cell together with calcium, and rapid depolarisation occurs giving phase 0 of the action potential (Fig. 2.7a). Repolarisation — the process by which the cell returns to its resting state — then begins, with a partial decline of the electrical potential (to about $+10$ mV). This is thought to be due to the negative chloride ion entering the cell, in addition to the inward Na^+ current being inactivated. Phase 1 of the action potential results.

Slowing of repolarisation results in a plateau — phase 2 of the action potential — which may allow for the sustained contraction of cardiac muscle. In phase 3, repolarisation speeds up: K^+ moves out of the cell more quickly and inactivation of the slow inward calcium current occurs. During phase 4 the sodium pump is reinstated. The resting myocardial cells await a further stimulus.

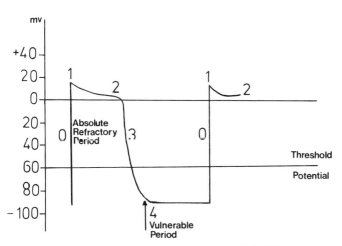

Fig. 2.7a   The phases of the action potential of the myocardial cells.

Action Potential of Pacemaker Cells

The action potential of the pacemaker cells is different from that of normal myocardial cells.

Pacemaker cells initiate the impulses for the heart — hence in phase 4 they do not wait to be stimulated from another source but display the property of slow diastolic depolarisation. Due to a slow influx of Na^+ during diastole, the cells become less negative on the inside and reach threshold potential producing the impulse which is conducted to the myocardial cells. For this reason, pacemaker cells are said to have an unstable resting stage (Fig. 2.7b). The cell which depolarises first will go on to depolarise all the cells of the heart.

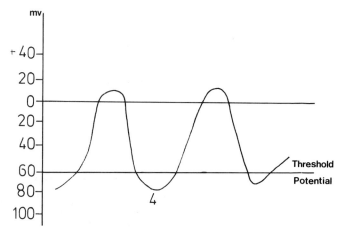

Fig. 2.7b   The phases of the action potential of the pacemaker cells.

Refractory Period

The absolute refractory period extends from the onset of depolarisation to approximately -50 to -60 mV of the repolarisation phase. During this time no other stimulus, regardless of strength, will produce an action potential. Immediately following the absolute refractory period, there exists a period of 'relative refractoriness', during which a strong impulse may result in an action potential. A vulnerable period follows this when even a relatively weak impulse may initiate an action potential (Fig. 2.7a).

The Cardiac Cycle

The cardiac cycle is the result of a series of electrical and mechanical events occurring in the heart. One complete cardiac cycle occurs about 70 times every minute; each cycle lasts approximately 0·8 of a second. The periods of contraction (systole) and relaxation (diastole) usually each last about 0·4 of a second, although diastolic time shortens with increasing heart rate (Fig. 2.8). The left side of the heart operates at much higher pressures than the right, but the action of the two sides is very similar.

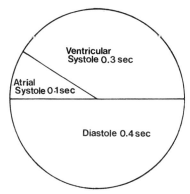

Fig. 2.8   The cardiac cycle.

When the pressure in the atria becomes greater than that in the ventricles, the AV valves open and blood flows from the atria to the ventricles. As the ventricles fill, the cusps of the tricuspid and mitral valves float upwards. The atria depolarise; the impulse is slowed down in the AV node to allow the atria time to contract. With atrial contraction, the AV valves are again forced open and ventricular filling is increased by one-sixth. The atria begin to relax and ventricular depolarisation and contraction occur. This results in ventricular pressure rising above atrial pressure and the AV valves closing completely.

Ventricular pressure continues to rise due to increased wall tension, although the volume of blood in the ventricles remains the same — the period of isovolumetric contraction. Eventually, ventricular pressure rises above that in the pulmonary artery (PA) and aorta, and their valves open as blood is ejected into them.

When pressure in the ventricles again falls below that in the PA and aorta, blood flow in these vessels ceases and the valves close.

The ventricles relax during the period of ventricular diastole and it is during this time that the AV valves open and the greatest part of ventricular filling occurs, the pressure in the atria again being slightly higher than that in the ventricles. The cardiac cycle is then repeated. The pressure wave-forms produced by these changes are shown in Fig. 2.9.

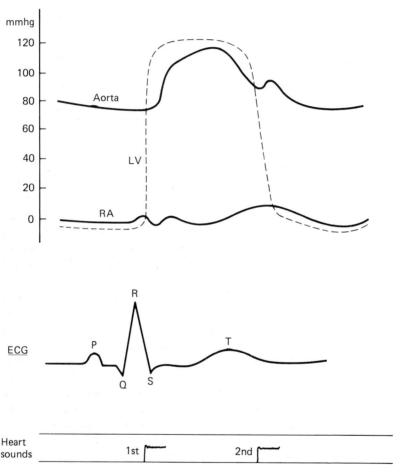

Fig. 2.9   Pressure waves in the aorta, right atrium and left ventricle.

Nerve Supply to the Heart

Although it is able to operate independently, the heart is supplied

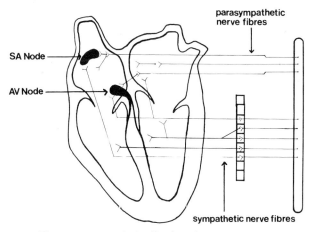

Fig. 2.10   The nerve supply to the heart.

with nerves from the autonomic nervous system, which influence the rate of impulse formation, the speed of conduction and the strength of the resulting cardiac contraction (Fig. 2.10). There are two different kinds of nerves making up the autonomic nervous system: the sympathetic and the parasympathetic nerves. The parasympathetic nerves are composed predominantly of fibres from the right and left vagus. The cardiac nerves originate in the cardiac centre of the medulla oblongata.

The fibres of the sympathetic nerves supply all of the atria and ventricles. Their stimulation tends to produce increased heart rate, increased speed of conduction and increased contractility of the myocardium. These responses are seen normally during exercise, emotion and stress. The fibres of the vagus nerves are located chiefly in the SA node, atrial muscle and AV node although they are also present in the ventricular myocardium. Vagus nerve stimulation causes reduction in heart rate and force of contraction and decreased speed of conduction through the AV node.

Pressure changes in the aorta and carotid arteries also influence heart rate and contractility. Sensory fibres extend from pressure sensitive receptors called baroreceptors in the aortic arch and carotid sinus to the vasomotor centre in the medulla which regulates the rate of nerve impulses. These impulses are conveyed to the heart by the sympathetic nerves and the cardiac branches of the vagus. The sensory impulses from the aortic arch are relayed through the vagus nerve and those from the carotid sinus via the

glossopharyngeal nerve. Both nerves send impulses to the vasomotor centre. Increased pressure is sensed by the baroreceptors
with the reflex effect of decreasing the rate and force of cardiac
contraction. This effect can be produced clinically by performing
carotid sinus massage. Decreased pressure has the opposite effect.

THE CORONARY CIRCULATION

The heart is supplied with oxygenated blood by the right and left
coronary arteries which arise from the sinuses of Valsalva of the
aorta, situated just above its exit from the LV. The elastic pockets
of the sinuses of Valsalva ensure a good coronary blood flow,
which is at its maximum during diastole. The main venous
drainage from the heart is by the coronary sinus into the RA but
numerous other smaller cardiac veins also drain the heart.

The Left Coronary Artery

The source of the left coronary artery is in the left sinus of Valsalva
of the aorta, just above the aortic valve (Fig. 2.11). After 2–3 cm it
divides into two branches called:

1.　the left anterior descending (LAD) coronary artery.
2.　the circumflex coronary artery.

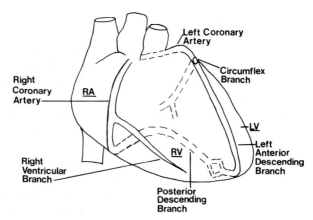

Fig. 2.11　The coronary arteries.

The LAD coronary artery extends inferiorly towards the apex of the heart in the anterior sulcus between the right and left ventricles. The diagonal branches of the LAD coronary artery supply the anterior LV wall and the septal branches supply the ventricular septum.

Myocardial infarction is the result of severe narrowing or occlusion of one or more coronary arteries. This usually occurs due to atherosclerosis which builds up over a period of years. The site of infarction depends on which coronary artery is involved. Occlusion of the LAD results in anterior myocardial infarction involving the antero-septal and/or antero-lateral LV wall (Fig. 2.12). It may affect the right and left bundle branches and result in disturbances of impulse conduction.

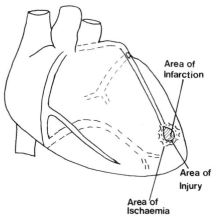

Fig. 2.12 An anterior myocardial infarction.

The circumflex coronary artery arises from the main left coronary artery and passes in the sulcus between the LA and the LV under the left atrial appendage. It gives off a varying number of left marginal branches and often terminates at the crux on the back of the heart in an anastomosis with the right coronary artery. However, the circumflex artery may descend between the ventricles at the back of the heart in a dominant left coronary artery system. The circumflex artery supplies the lateral and posterior aspects of the LV and its branches also supply the LA. Occlusion of this artery usually results in lateral LV or posterior myocardial infarction (Fig. 2.13). However, obstruction of a dominant circumflex coronary artery may cause inferior infarction.

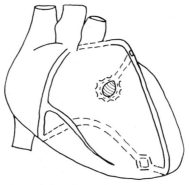

Fig. 2.13 Occlusion of the circumflex coronary artery resulting in posterior left ventricular wall infarction.

The Right Coronary Artery

The right coronary artery (RCA) originates from the right or anterior sinus of Valsalva, and courses along the atrioventricular sulcus between the RA and RV. Small branches which supply the SA node and pulmonary trunk arise within the first few centimetres. Then a more major branch, the right ventricular branch, arises to supply the anterior surface of the RV. The main RCA continues round the right border of the heart, still in the AV sulcus, and gives off further branches to the RA and RV. At the crux of the heart, the RCA usually turns downwards to become the posterior descending coronary artery. It descends between the right and left ventricles in the interventricular groove, supplying

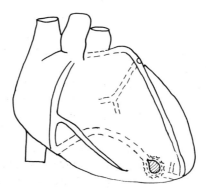

Fig. 2.14 Occlusion of the right coronary artery resulting in inferior left ventricular wall infarction.

the inferior surface of the LV. This is described as a dominant right coronary artery system and occurs in 50–80% of the population. Normally, the branches of the RCA supply the RA, SA node, AV node and bundle, and the RV and inferior aspect of the LV. Occlusion of this artery may cause right ventricular infarction (rare), or more commonly inferior infarction of the LV (Fig. 2.14). AV conduction disturbances of rhythm are common with RCA occlusion. However, these are often transient and resolve as recovery occurs.

The major coronary arteries have a subepicardial course and may be partly embedded in fatty tissue. The terminal branches of these arteries run at right angles into the muscle mass.

Anastomoses

Normally, many small anastomoses exist between the coronary arteries but these are relatively unimportant in health. However, in the presence of myocardial ischaemia, they enlarge providing collateral blood supply to the affected area.

Oxygen

A considerable amount of oxygen is extracted from the blood in the coronary arteries by the myocardium. The oxygen concentration of blood entering the RA via the coronary sinus is much less than that entering it from the superior and inferior vena cavae.

Dominant Coronary Artery Systems

The RCA is usually the dominant artery — at the crux of the heart it becomes the posterior descending coronary artery. Less often, the circumflex artery is dominant in that it becomes the posterior descending coronary artery at the crux of the heart. In some patients, the right and left coronary arteries both reach the crux and descend together down the posterior interventricular groove. This is described as a 'balanced' coronary artery system.

Indeed the coronary arteries are very variable. The LAD artery may occasionally cross the apex and proceed upward in the posterior interventricular groove. Sometimes, the RCA divides to become the posterior descending coronary artery and continues in the atrioventricular groove to supply much of the lateral aspect of the LV.

Further reading

Andreoli K.G., Hunn-Fowkes V., Zipes D.P., Wallace A.G. (1979). Anatomy and physiology of the heart. In *Comprehensive Cardiac Care: a Text for Nurses, Physicians and Other Health Practitioners*, 4th edn., pp.1–7. St. Louis: The C.V. Mosby Company.

Conover M.B. (1980). Anatomy and physiology of the heart and electrophysiology of the normal heart. In *Understanding Electrocardiography, Physiological and Interpretive Concepts*, 3rd edn., pp.1–12 and 13–22. St. Louis: The C.V. Mosby Company.

Navaratnam V. (1975). Anatomy of the Heart and Cardiac Excitability and Electrical Activity. In *The Human Heart and Circulation*, 1st edn., pp.5–27 and 56–75. London, New York, San Francisco: Academic Press.

Ochsner J.L., Mills N.L. (1978). Anatomy: Correlated Angiographic and Surgical Findings. In *Coronary Artery Surgery*, 1st edn., pp. 20–54. Philadelphia: Lea and Febiger.

Ross J.S., Wilson K.J.W. (1981). The Circulatory System. In *Foundations of Anatomy and Physiology*, 5th edn., pp.58–62. Edinburgh: Churchill Livingstone.

Thompson D.R. (1982). The heart. In *Cardiac Nursing*, 1st edn., pp. 7–43. London: Baillière Tindall.

3

The Electrocardiogram

BASIC ECG MONITORING IN THE CCU

The original concept of coronary care was to prevent death from cardiac arrest. Later attention was directed to the early detection and treatment of arrhythmias which not only caused cardiac arrest but also those which led to cardiac failure and syncope. Techniques for monitoring have improved over the years and are now more sophisticated, providing valuable information which influences the management of the patient.

The Bedside Oscilloscope

This displays the ECG at the patient's bedside. The tracing can be relayed to the central monitoring station. Controls on the oscilloscope can adjust the size and brightness of the picture. A digital display of the patient's heart rate can be seen at the side of the trace. Incorporated into the system is an alarm which is both audible and visible. This is activated by a heart rate meter which can be adjusted according to the needs of the patient. The usual range is between 50–150 beats/min. If the heart rate changes to a level outside this range, the alarm system is triggered. In many models this activates a direct write-out at the central console, providing a permanent record of the patient's ECG. Recordings can be taken for a selected length of time or can be continuous, as is necessary during a cardiac arrest.

The Central Console

The central console consists of a large oscilloscope capable of displaying ECGs of all the patients in the coronary care unit, allowing their continuous surveillance (Fig. 3.1). A memory facility may be incorporated into the system.

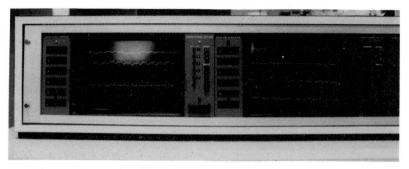

Fig. 3.1 The central console.

THE ELECTROCARDIOGRAM

Cardiac muscle generates electrical currents which can be detected by electrodes attached to the skin. These in turn are attached to a recording instrument which displays the graphic trace of the ECG.

Application of Electrodes

The aim when applying electrodes is to achieve a narrow stable base line without noise (distortion) and of sufficient 'R' wave amplitude. There is no universally agreed position for electrodes and thus the sites of adhesion vary from unit to unit.

The skin should be shaved if the chest is hairy. Bony protruberances should be avoided. The chosen sites should be clean and dry. Alcohol can be used to clean the skin and the areas should be dried briskly with gauze before applying the electrode. The pre-gelled electrode is attached to the skin by running the finger around the edge of the electrode to produce firm adhesion. Poor application technique may produce an unsatisfactory trace. Dry electrodes or broken leads may also cause this problem which may result in repeated activation of the alarm system.

Occasionally skin irritation may be caused by the electrodes but in normal circumstances it is not necessary to change the electrodes daily.

Telemetric Monitoring

Telemetry is a convenient way of monitoring the cardiac rhythm during the mobilisation of patients as there are no direct leads to the monitor. Electrodes are attached to the chest in the normal way and these in turn are connected to a small portable battery operated transmitter. The radio frequency signals are then received by the central monitor and the ECG is displayed on its screen.

Electrophysiology

To interpret the ECG, it is necessary to understand the electrophysiological principles of the heart as described in Chapter 2. However, a brief outline is also included here.

Polarisation

The inside of the resting cardiac cell is electrically negative compared with the outside, i.e. the cell is 'polarised' (Fig. 3.2). This situation arises because the extracellular concentration of positively charged sodium ions greatly exceeds the intracellular concentration. Sodium ions are prevented from diffusing into the cells down the concentration gradient by the action of the 'sodium pump', an energy requiring metabolic process. In contrast, the intracellular potassium concentration is greater than the extracellular concentration although these ions are quantitatively much less important determinants of the overall electrical state. An ECG recorded during the resting phase would show no deviation from the isoelectric base line.

Depolarisation

When the resting cardiac cell is stimulated, there is a change in the cell membrane permeability to sodium (as well as calcium) ions which flood into the cell. This is known as 'depolarisation' and as a result the inside of the cell becomes electrically positive compared

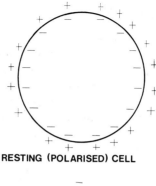

RESTING (POLARISED) CELL

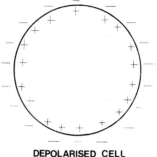

DEPOLARISED CELL

Fig. 3.2   The electrical charges on a polarised and a depolarised myocardial cell.

to the outside (Fig. 3.2). Rapid depolarisation occurs until an equilibrium exists and sodium ions cease to enter the cell. An electrical current is generated by depolarisation, which spreads to neighbouring polarised cells causing them in turn to depolarise. The spread of these impulses is recorded on the ECG as the P and QRS deflections. The P wave represents atrial depolarisation while ventricular depolarisation causes the QRS complex.

Repolarisation

During repolarisation the cells are restored to their former electrical state as sodium ions are once again pumped out of the cell. On the ECG, the T wave represents ventricular repolarisation. Atrial repolarisation is not seen on the ECG as it is masked by the QRS.

Automaticity (Diastolic Depolarisation)

Some specialised cells (for example, those in the sinus node, part of the atria, the AV junction and Purkinje system) are able to fire spontaneously without any external stimulation.

The sinus node normally has the fastest firing rate and is thus the pacemaker of the heart. The rate is usually 60–100 beats/min. However, if one of the other areas increases its rate of discharge, or the sinus node slows, then the faster pacemaker will control the heart. The normal rhythm of the heart is called sinus rhythm.

Cardiac Vector

A vector is a term used to describe an electrical force which has both magnitude and direction. Diagrammatically this may be depicted by an arrow, the angle of which shows direction, and the length of which shows magnitude.

Depolarisation goes through a sequence, the direction of which is constantly changing. As vectors of equal magnitude going in opposite directions cancel each other out, total activity can be represented by single vectors, known as instantaneous vectors. A vector which occurs in the cardiac cycle is known as a cardiac vector.

Conduction of the Heart

The conduction system of the heart is described in Chapter 2. The impulse normally arises in the sinus node which is situated near to the entrance of the superior vena cava. It then spreads across the atria causing them to contract. The impulse reaches the AV node, located close to the tricuspid valve in the right atrial wall and from here it passes down the bundle of His and into the right and left bundle branches before entering the Purkinje network and pro-ducing ventricular contraction. (See Fig. 3.3.)

THE STANDARD 12 LEAD ELECTROCARDIOGRAM

The 12 lead ECG is of paramount importance in the diagnosis of heart disease. In 1903 William Einthoven of Leyden invented the electrocardiograph. At this time it was realised that the heart beat

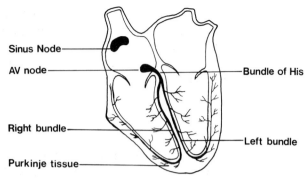

Fig. 3.3   The conduction system of the heart.

probably coincided with electrical charges but these could not be measured on a galvanometer (an instrument which detects small electrical currents). Using the principle that the heart is in the centre of a magnetic field, Einthoven stretched a thread of silver-coated quartz between the poles of a powerful magnet set at right angles to this field. The thread was connected to two pads soaked in salt solution and placed on the limbs of the patients — as far away from the heart as possible. When the magnetic field was turned on, the thread was observed to pulsate with each beat. Then, by taking a series of photographs, Einthoven was able to document a graphic recording of the electrical changes of the

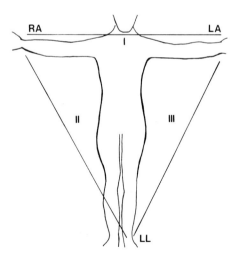

Fig. 3.4   The Einthoven Triangle.

heart. He described the three peripheral electrodes as forming an equilateral triangle with the heart at the centre. The right leg is used as the ground electrode. The triaxial figure is based on Einthoven's triangle and the assumption that leads I, II and III are equidistant from the heart. (See Fig. 3.4.)

The Bipolar Leads

These are attached to the limbs and measure the difference in electrical potential between two recording sites. The leads are as follows:

Lead I = Left arm (positive) + right arm (negative).
Lead II = Left leg (positive) + right arm (negative).
Lead III = Left leg (positive) + left arm (negative).

The Unipolar Leads

These are called the 'V' leads and consist of three limb leads (Fig. 3.5) and six precordial chest leads. Two electrodes are again used but one is an exploring electrode recording potential changes in the leads while the other is an indifferent lead and registers a potential of zero.

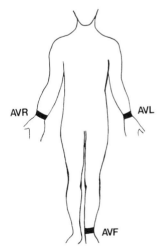

Fig. 3.5   The unipolar limb leads.

Lead aVR = Right arm (positive) + indifferent lead (negative).
Lead aVL = Left arm (positive) + indifferent lead (negative).
Lead aVF = Left foot (positive) + indifferent lead (negative).

These unipolar leads combined with the standard limb leads form the hexaxial reference system.

The Unipolar Chest Leads

An electrode is placed on six points on the precordium as follows (Fig. 3.6):

V_1 = The fourth intercostal space right of the sternum.
V_2 = The fourth intercostal space just left of the sternum.
V_3 = Midway between V_2–V_4.
V_4 = The fifth intercostal space in the mid-clavicular line.
V_5 = Left anterior axillary line at the same horizontal line as V_4.
V_6 = Left mid-axillary line at the same horizontal line as lead V_4.

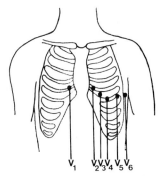

Fig. 3.6   The electrode position of the precordial leads.

Sometimes other recording sites are used. These include V_7 and V_8 which extend laterally. Alternatively the electrodes may be placed on a higher intercostal space. These sites may be helpful when the site of infarction is obscure. Marking of the chest facilitates identical electrodes positioning for serial ECGs.

Recording the Electrocardiograph

The techniques of recording should be explained to the patient. Reassurance is given regarding the safety of the procedure. The patient's chest is shaved if necessary and watches and jewellery should be removed as they can cause electrical interference. The patient should be as relaxed as possible to avoid muscle tremor. Electrode cream is applied to the appropriate sites and the electrodes attached. Before actual ECG recording takes place, checks should be made to ensure that standardisation is correct and that the isoelectric baseline is horizontal.

The Recording Paper

The paper is marked with both horizontal and vertical lines (Fig. 3.7). The lines are 1 mm apart. Every fifth line is more heavily marked than the others. The horizontal lines measure the amplitude. The vertical lines are representative of time duration. Each line represents 0·04 sec, while the fifth more heavily marked line represents 0·2 sec if the paper speed is 25 mm/sec. The electrocardiogram is described as a series of negative and positive deflections. Positive deflections rise above the baseline and negative deflections descend below it. The deflections are identified by the

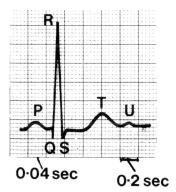

Fig. 3.7   The recording paper.

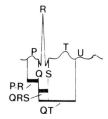

Fig. 3.8   ECG intervals.

letters PQRST and U (chosen at random) (Fig. 3.8). Positive deflections are caused by electrical currents flowing towards the electrode and negative deflections by movement away from the electrode. Those currents running at right angles to the electrode result in equiphasic deflections.

The P Wave

The P wave represents the spread of electrical activity across the atria. The normal P wave can be positive, negative or biphasic depending on which lead is being recorded. It is normally inverted in AVR. The amplitude of the P wave should not exceed 3 mm. The PR interval is measured from the beginning of the P wave to the beginning of the QRS complex and measures between 0·12–0·20 sec in adults. There is an isoelectric line between the P wave and QRS complex. This is the interval between the end of atrial depolarisation and the beginning of ventricular depolarisation. A shortened PR interval may be an indication of Wolff–Parkinson–White syndrome. A long PR interval signifies conduction disorders.

The QRS Complex

This represents ventricular depolarisation. The components of the QRS complex vary depending on the lead of the electrocardiogram being recorded. The Q wave is any initial negative deflection preceeding an R wave. The R wave is the positive deflection. Even if a second positive deflection is recorded, this is still known as an R wave.

The S wave is any negative deflection following an R wave. A QS complex denotes a totally negative deflection (Fig. 3.9). The normal QRS complex is no wider than 0·10 sec. A broad QRS complex may signify bundle branch block. The initial depolarisation starts in the left side of the interventricular septum, activating it from left to right. The electrocardiogram will therefore show an upward deflection or small r wave in the right chest leads. A small q wave or downward deflection is normally seen over the left chest leads. Although depolarisation of the ventricles is simultaneous and spreads through the free walls from the endocardium to epicardium, it is the left ventricle which is the most dominant because of its size. The resultant vector is therefore from right to

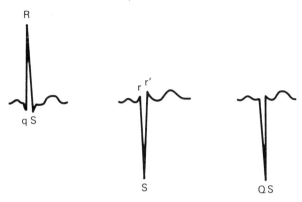

Fig. 3.9   The components of the QRS complex.

left. An electrode over the right chest leads will show a deep S wave and over the left ventricle will record an R wave. Thus, to summarise, in the right ventricular leads V_1 and V_2, an rS complex will be seen; over the left ventricular leads V_5 and V_6, a qR complex is normal (see Fig. 3.10). Small deflections are often denoted by small letters whereas capital letters usually represent larger deflections.

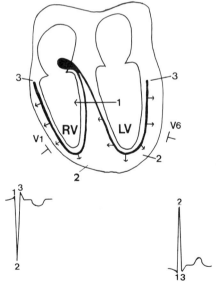

Fig. 3.10   Normal ventricular depolarisation: 1. from left to right across the septum; 2. depolarisation of main ventricle walls (endocardium to epicardium); 3. base of ventricle walls.

The ST Segment

The ST segment curves upward from the isoelectric line. The normal limit is less than 1·0 mm on the ECG. Elevation of the ST segment is suggestive of myocardial infarction and Prinzmetal angina, while ST depression may indicate ischaemia. Depression of the terminal part of the ST segment may be found on the ECG of patients on digitalis therapy.

The J point is to be found at the junction of the S wave and ST segment. This becomes exaggerated in hypothermia and is called the J wave.

The T Wave

This represents the recovery period or repolarisation of the ventricles. The T wave is normally upright in leads I, II, V_3–V_6. It is always inverted in AVR. In other leads it may be upright or inverted. In the precordial leads the T wave should not exceed 10 mm in height while in the standard leads the normal maximum is 5 mm. Inverted T waves may suggest ischaemia. Tall peaked waves may indicate hyperkalaemia.

The U Wave

The U wave is a small voltage wave following the T wave and little is known about it. It may increase in magnitude if hypokalaemia is present. An inverted U wave is always abnormal.

Interpreting the Electrocardiogram

The heart rate may be calcuated by using one of the specially designed rulers or by using the ECG graph paper. If the ventricular rate is regular, and the paper speed is 25 mm/sec, divide the number of small squares on the paper between the R waves into 1500. The larger squares can also be used by dividing into 300. If the rhythm is irregular, however, count the number of R waves in 6 seconds and multiply by 10.

Rhythm Analysis

1. Note if P waves are present and whether their relationship with the QRS complex is constant.

2. Note how many P waves there are to each QRS complex.
3. Measure the PR interval. This should not be less than 0·12 sec or greater than 0·20 sec.
4. Look at the QRS complex. A broad complex is an indication of bundle branch block.
5. Finally, look at each lead systematically for any deviation from the normal electrocardiograph.

The Mean Axis

The electrical activity or depolarisation is represented by vectors (see p. 27). The average or dominant direction of these vectors is known as the mean QRS axis. The hexaxial system (see p. 30) is used to obtain the mean QRS axis. This is a combination of Einthoven's triangle plus the three unipolar limb leads (Fig. 3.11).

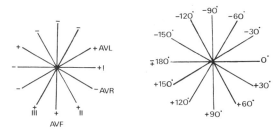

Fig. 3.11   The triaxial and hexaxial reference systems.

The normal range of the QRS axis is 0° to +90°. A right axis deviation lies between +90° and +180°. A left axis deviation lies between −30° and −120° (0° to −30° can be equivocal). Variations in the axis may result from ventricular hypertrophy, the electrical position of the heart or developing conduction defects (see Chapter 7).

To Determine the Mean QRS Axis

First, look for the lead with the most equiphasic deflection, that is of equal amplitude above and below the line. Second, find the lead which is at right angles to the above lead. This lead should register the greatest deflection. Note whether the deflection is positive or negative. The axis will be directed parallel to this lead. Figure 3.12 shows an ECG within normal limits.

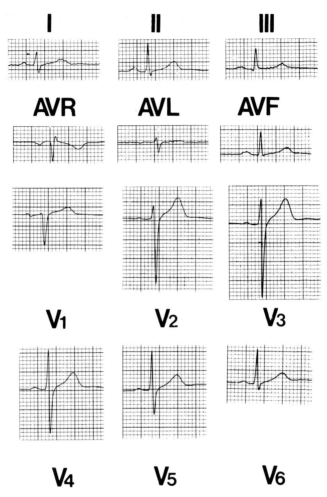

Fig. 3.12 This is an example of a normal ECG. The axis is normal.

Further Reading

Andreoli K.G., Hunn-Fowkes V., Zipes D.P., Wallace A.F. (1977). *Comprehensive Cardiac Care*, pp.77–115. St. Louis: The C.V. Mosby Company.

Julian D.G. (1983). *Cardiology*, 4th edn., pp.28–48. London: Ballière Tindall.

Meltzer L.E., Pinneo R., Kitchell J.R. (1977). *Intensive Coronary Care*, 3rd edn., pp.121–137. Bowie, Md.: The Charles Press Publishers.

Rowlands D.J. (1982). *Understanding the Electrocardiogram*. Maccles-field: Imperial Chemical Industries.

Schamroth L. (1977). *An Introduction to Electrocardiography*, 5th edn. Oxford: Blackwell.

Thompson D.R. (1982). *Cardiac Nursing*, 1st edn., pp.44–64. London: Ballière Tindall.

4

Angina

ATHEROSCLEROSIS

Atherosclerosis is a common disease affecting the coronary arteries. Over a period of years, cholesterol and other substances are laid down as atheromatous plaque along the intimal lining of the arteries, thus narrowing the passages and reducing the blood flow through them. When the oxygen supply to the myocardium is insufficient for its needs, the symptoms of coronary artery disease may be encountered.

Several factors are thought to be related to the rate at which atherosclerosis develops: a diet high in animal fat content, smoking and hypertension. Emotional stress, obesity, a sedentary life-style and an aggressive personality are also thought to contribute.

Men between the ages of 45 and 60 are affected twice as commonly as women in this age group. Over the age of 60, the incidence is approximately the same in both sexes.

Angina

The most common symptom of myocardial ischaemia is angina pectoris. This characteristic chest pain may be due to metabolites produced as a result of inadequate oxygen supply (anaerobic metabolism). The primary mechanisms causing angina are: fixed atheromatous lesions, coronary artery spasm, and a combination of these two mechanisms. However, it may also occur as a result of other conditions. Arrhythmias may cause decreased coronary artery perfusion without significant coronary artery disease. Severe anaemia results in decreased oxygen carrying ability of the blood, thus oxygen supply to the myocardium may be insufficient to meet its needs. Aortic valve disease often increases the work load of the myocardium without increasing its blood supply. Hypothyroidism and hyperthyroidism may also be associated with angina.

Characteristics of Angina Pectoris

There are certain recognised characteristics of the pain of angina:

1. site
2. nature
3. relationship to exercise
4. duration
5. response to glyceryl trinitrate.

Site

The pain is often described as occurring centrally under the sternum although it may also be felt on either side of the chest, particularly on the left. It may radiate to the neck, jaw, back or arms. Often it affects one or two of these areas only. It may present as tingling or numbness in the arms or fingers.

The nature of the pain

The nature of the pain is that of pressure or tightness in the chest, often described as a heavy weight or a tight constricting band. Some patients experience a choking feeling, others the sensation of toothache in the gums. Still others describe only a feeling of vague discomfort and are reluctant to describe it as pain.

Relationship to exercise

Generally, the pain of angina comes on during exercise, as this increases heart work and thereby increases the myocardial demand for oxygen. It is invariably relieved by rest. Large meals, cold and windy weather and emotional crises are known to precipitate attacks. Sometimes nocturnal angina may waken a patient from sleep.

Duration

Attacks of angina are usually short — a maximum of two or three minutes. If an attack lasts longer than 15 minutes, sustained ischaemia results with possible destruction of the myocardium.

Response to glyceryl trinitrate

Glyceryl trinitrate (GTN) is often successful in relieving angina by dilating the coronary arteries, increasing coronary blood flow and decreasing venous return to the heart, thus reducing heart work. Sometimes GTN is used as a means of establishing the diagnosis. If the pain is unrelieved after the administration of two or three fresh GTN tablets, the diagnosis of angina pectoris must be in doubt.

Other Symptoms

Patients may describe other symptoms in association with the chest pain of angina. Breathlessness, sweating, flatulance, faintness, nausea, anxiety and a general feeling of uneasiness may be noticed. If chest pain is induced by an arrhythmia, palpitations may be felt before the pain occurs.

Stable and Unstable Angina

A patient can be described as having stable angina when stress or exertion predictably induce pain. It will be easily and quickly relieved by rest and GTN. If the angina appears on minimal exertion or rest, and the attacks are more severe and difficult to control, then the situation is one of unstable angina. Some authors describe the severe and longer-lasting episodes of angina as pre-infarction syndrome since these may precede myocardial infarction.

Making the Diagnosis of Angina

In making the diagnosis of angina, an accurate history is of utmost importance. Many patients will describe pain which has several of the characteristic features.

Physical examination may reveal risk factors of atherosclerosis. It may also reveal abnormal heart sounds and evidence of other diseases which may induce or exacerbate angina. However, it is important to appreciate that a normal examination does not exclude a diagnosis of angina.

INVESTIGATIONS

Several investigations are of value in establishing a diagnosis of angina:

1. the ECG
2. the exercise test
3. coronary arteriography
4. thallium scanning.

The ECG

The ECG of a patient with angina may be normal between attacks of pain. T wave changes alone are not diagnostic of ischaemic heart disease, since a number of other conditions may affect this part of the ECG complex (Table 4.1). The majority of patients experiencing angina produce some ECG changes during an attack. Should the ST segment become depressed, either in a horizontal or sloping fashion, this is very suggestive of ischaemic heart disease (Fig. 4.1a and 4.1b). Angina due to coronary artery spasm (Prinzmetal angina) produces a characteristic ECG change of ST elevation during pain (Fig. 4.1c). Occasionally, a resting abnormality may transiently disappear during an episode of angina, only to return when the patient is painfree. This 'pseudo-normalisation' of the ECG should be regarded as a significant finding. Thus the coronary care nurse must understand the importance of obtaining ECGs during the patient's chest pain, in addition to when he is pain free.

Exercise Testing

Exercise tests are often performed to assess the ability of the heart to respond to increased demand for oxygen. An established

TABLE 4.1
Conditions which may affect the ST segment and mimic ischaemia of the myocardium

Anxiety
Heavy meals
Hyperventilation
Smoking
Iced Drinks
Reduced blood pressure
Changes in body position
Electrolyte disturbances
Left ventricular diastolic overload and hypertrophy
Acute pericarditis and myocarditis
Head injury
Digoxin and quinidine administration
Sympathetic nervous system dysfunction
Wolff–Parkinson–White syndrome

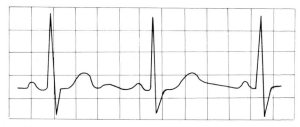

Fig. 4.1a   The normal ECG of a patient at rest.

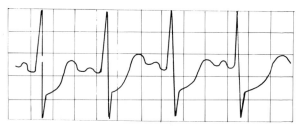

Fig. 4.1b   ST segment depression and increased heart rate occurring on exercise and associated with angina.

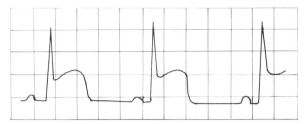

Fig. 4.1c   The ECG of a patient with Prinzmetal angina shows ST elevation during an episode of chest pain.

protocol such as the Bruce protocol is used, the levels of exercise being increased at set times (Table 4.2). Careful recordings of blood pressure, heart rate and symptoms are made before, during and after exercise. An ECG is recorded continuously throughout the test. Should horizontal ST depression of 1 mm or more occur related to exercise, this is a positive result (Fig. 4.2). The time from starting the exercise until the onset of symptoms is of significance regarding prognosis.

Exercise tests are not without difficulties, however, since false positives and negatives do occur. Arrhythmias may arise and cause early discontinuation of the test, thus preventing accurate interpretation. Exercise tests have a small risk of serious complications. They should be performed in a safe, controlled environment with emergency equipment and drugs close at hand and a doctor in attendance. More recently, limited exercise tests are being performed as soon as seven days after myocardial infarction.

TABLE 4.2
Bruce Protocol

Each stage for 3 minutes	
Stage I	1.7 mph at 10% gradient
II	2.5 mph at 12% gradient
III	3.4 mph at 14% gradient
IV	4.2 mph at 16% gradient
V	5.0 mph at 18% gradient
VI	5.5 mph at 20% gradient
VII	6.0 mph at 22% gradient

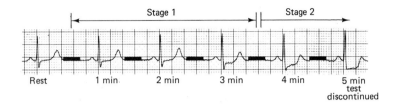

Fig. 4.2   The ECG of a patient with a positive exercise test. Test followed Bruce Protocol (Table 4.2). The first complex was recorded during the pre-exercise resting period. Complexes are shown after 1, 2, 3, 4 and 5 minutes of exercise.

Coronary Arteriography

Coronary arteriography is performed when a definite diagnosis of coronary atherosclerosis, and the extent of it, is required. This degree of detail is necessary if the patient is a candidate for coronary artery bypass surgery. Specifically designed catheters are available for entering both the right and left coronary arteries. Contrast medium can be injected through these to outline the vessels. Cine-angiograms are then taken as permanent records to be analysed later.

Patients considered for this invasive procedure are usually those with:

1. unstable angina.
2. stable angina which is unresponsive to medical treatment.
3. aortic valve disease and secondary angina.
4. frequent admissions to hospital with chest pain but the diagnosis of ischaemia unconfirmed by ECGs and cardiac enzymes.
5. careers in which safety factors are of great importance such as drivers, air pilots and others.

Coronary arteriography can be associated with complications such as life threatening arrhythmias, myocardial infarction or sudden death. Adverse reactions to the radio-opaque dye may also occur. For these reasons, the procedure is performed in a 'safe' environment and mortality is low — between 0·1 and 0·5%.

Thallium Scanning

Thallium scanning is another procedure which can help to diagnose myocardial ischaemia. It involves the intravenous injection of the radio-isotope thallium. This is transported to the heart, where it is taken up by the cells. Areas of poor perfusion — called cold areas — do not take up the radio-isotope as readily as parts of good perfusion. Thus ischaemic areas can be identified on the scan.

Differential diagnosis

There are several conditions in which chest pain may mimic that of angina pectoris (Table 4.3). Indeed any of these may be present in addition to angina. However, a careful history and thorough examination should eliminate most. Inflammation of the costochondral junctions (Tietze's syndrome) and muscular aches and pains of the chest wall are often associated with tenderness, inflammation and swelling. The pain of pericarditis is usually worse on inspiration and movement.

The symptoms of lung disorders should be distinguishable from angina. However, the pain of oesophageal spasm and reflux oesophagitis may mimic angina very closely and may be very difficult to differentiate from cardiac pain.

TABLE 4.3
Differential Diagnosis of Angina Pectoris

Tietze's syndrome
Muscular pains of the chest wall
Pericarditis
Pneumothorax
Asthmatic attacks
Airways obstruction
Oesophageal spasm, reflex oesophagitis
Cholecystitis
Peptic ulcer
Dissecting aneurysm
Hyperventilation and anxiety

Cholecystitis may produce chest discomfort but attacks are too prolonged to be angina and are often associated with abdominal tenderness and nausea. Attacks of pain from peptic ulcers are also prolonged. The pain of a dissecting aneurysm may mimic that of angina. T wave changes on the ECG can be produced by conditions such as anxiety, hyperventilation and hypertension without underlying coronary artery disease, making the diagnosis more difficult.

TREATMENT OF ANGINA

There are several possible forms of treatment for angina and the choice depends primarily on the nature and severity of the patient's symptoms.

After the diagnosis is confirmed, reassurance is very important as the term 'angina' induces anxiety in most sufferers. Advice should be given about reduction or elimination of risk factors with particular attention to weight loss and cessation of smoking. Information must also be given about general life-style factors which are likely to precipitate attacks of chest pain, how to avoid these factors and how to pace daily life so that fitness is preserved without sudden bursts of strenuous physical or emotional effort. Advice about the use of GTN is necessary — its storage, when and how it should be taken, its anticipated speed of action and possible side-effects. Headaches should be anticipated initially when taking GTN but these will diminish with usage. Patients should be encouraged to renew their supply regularly as the potency of the medication's action diminishes with age. It is illegal for people with angina to pursue certain careers. Public service and heavy goods vehicle licences will not be renewed after a diagnosis of angina has been made, so advice about a change of employment is necessary. These patients in particular need psychological support and may benefit from the help of the rehabilitation officer.

If angina is due to a cause unrelated to atherosclerosis, the symptoms may disappear when the appropriate treatment for the condition is given.

Drug Therapy

Many drugs are currently used in the treatment of angina pectoris.

Glyceryl Trinitrate

GTN is very widely used. The sublingual tablet can be taken to relieve an attack or prophylactically in anticipation of exercise which might precipitate pain. GTN dilates the coronary arteries and decreases venous return to the heart. Its side-effects include headaches, facial flushing and hypotension which may be sufficiently severe to produce syncope on occasions. Sublingual tablets have a short life of about eight weeks and must be stored in a tightly-capped brown glass bottle away from direct light, or more rapid deterioration will occur. Patients may be anxious about taking too many of these tablets and must be reassured that they are not addictive.

In addition to the sublingual preparation, glyceryl trinitrate is available in a chewable tablet, an oral preparation (normal and sustained release), an oral spray, topical forms and as an intravenous injection. Amyl nitrite is available for inhalation.

Beta Adrenoceptor Blocking Agents (Beta blockers)

This group of drugs is used either alone or in combination with trinitrates and calcium antagonists in the treatment of angina pectoris. Their effect is to block the action of catecholamines on the beta receptors of the body. This results in a reduced heart rate and blood pressure. The negative inotropic effect of beta blockers means that cardiac contractility is decreased, reducing myocardial workload and oxygen consumption during stress. Cardioselective beta blockers act predominantly on the beta-1 receptors of the myocardium giving the above results. Metoprolol, atenolol and acebutolol fall into this category. Propranolol, nadolol, oxprenolol and sotalol act also on the beta-2 receptors of the bronchial and vascular smooth muscle. Bronchospasm and cold peripheries are common side-effects of these non-cardioselective beta blockers.

Calcium Antagonists

The calcium antagonists verapamil and niphedipine are used in the treatment of arrhythmias and angina. Verapamil has a potent slowing effect on the conduction of the atrioventricular node. It also dilates the coronary arteries and peripheral vessels. Niphedipine also dilates the coronary arteries and decreases peripheral resistance by relaxing the smooth muscle of the blood vessel walls. This reduces the afterload (resistance against which the heart has to pump), but hypotension and tachycardia may result. Calcium antagonists, particularly niphedipine, have proved to be of great benefit in the treatment of Prinzmetal angina.

The Intra Aortic Balloon Pump

When a patient has unstable angina which is refractory to medical treatment and he is a possible candidate for coronary artery bypass grafts, consideration may be given to the use of the intra aortic balloon pump, to stabilise the situation until coronary arteriography and surgery can be arranged (see Chapter 11).

Coronary Artery Bypass Grafts

Patients with severe atherosclerosis of the coronary vessels supplying the left ventricle, and those with severe symptoms unrelieved by medical treatment, may be considered for coronary artery bypass surgery if they are otherwise fit for this operation. The main objective of this surgery is to relieve the symptoms of angina. Large scale trials have shown that life expectancy may be increased following coronary artery bypass grafts in patients who have disease of the left main descending coronary artery or of all three major vessels. Coronary artery bypass surgery involves bypassing the narrowed sections of the coronary arteries. A saphenous vein graft from the leg is usually used, one end being attached to the aorta and the other to the coronary artery beyond the narrowed section. Multiple grafts can be inserted.

Coronary Angioplasty

Angioplasty of the coronary arteries is a recently developed technique which is becoming popular as a means of treating single vessel disease. It involves the insertion of a small balloon catheter into the coronary artery. Inflation of the balloon to flatten the narrowed area has proved to be successful and may achieve similar benefits in pain relief to coronary artery bypass surgery.

PROGNOSIS

The prognosis of patients with angina pectoris is variable. Some patients develop good collateral circulation and may be relatively symptom-free for long periods of time. Others again may have less widespread disease, but more severe symptoms.

Indeed many patients can lead fairly normal lives for many years. If angina is associated with diseases such as hypertension, cardiac failure or myocardial infarction, the prognosis is less favourable. Generally the prognosis is dependent upon the severity of atherosclerosis and the number of vessels involved.

Further Reading

Akhras F., Upward J., Stott R., Jackson G. (1982). Early exercise testing and coronary angiography after uncomplicated myocardial infarction. *British Medical Journal*; **284**:1293–1294.

Boyle R.M. (1981). Exercise testing in ischaemic heart disease. *British Journal of Hospital Medicine;* **21**:8–14.

Chaitman B.R., Rogers W.J., Davis K., *et al.* (1980). Operative Risk Factors in Patients with Left Main Coronary Artery Disease. *The New England Journal of Medicine;* **303**: 953–957.

Fox K.M. (1982). Exercise testing in the diagnosis of ischaemic heart disease. *British Medical Journal;* **284**:611–612.

Heller R.F., Jacobs H.S. (1978). Coronary heart disease in relation to age, sex and the menopause. *British Medical Journal*; **1**:472–474.

Heller R.F., Hayward D., Hobbs M.S.T. (1983). Decline in rate of death from ischaemic heart disease in the United Kingdom. *British Medical Journal;* **286**:260–262.

Irving J.B. (1982). Exercise Stress Testing. *Hospital Update;* **8**:171–183.

Julian D.G. (1983). Disease of the Coronary Arteries. In *Cardiology*, 4th edn., pp.125–162. London: Baillière Tindall.

Julian D.G., Matthews M.B. (1977). Diseases of the Cardiovascular System. In *Davidson's Principles and Practice of Medicine: a Textbook for Students and Doctors.* (Macleod, J., ed.) 12th edn., pp.171–247. Edinburgh: Churchill Livingstone.

Khosla T., Newcombe R.G., Campbell H. (1977). Who is at risk of a coronary? *British Medical Journal;* **1**:341–344.

Lewis B. (1980). Dietary prevention of ischaemic heart disease — a policy for the '80s. *British Medical Journal;* **281**:177–180.

Meltzer L.E., Pinneo R., Kitchell J.R. (1977). Coronary Heart Disease. In *Intensive Coronary Care: a manual for nurses*, 3rd edn., pp.1–12. Bowie, Md.: The Charles Press Publishers.

Miller D., Waters D.D., Warnica W., Szlachcic J., Kreeft J., Théroux P. (1981). Is Variant Angina the Coronary Manifestation of a Generalized Vasospastic Disorder? *The New England Journal of Medicine;* **304**:763–766.

Ockene I.S., Shay M.J., Alpert J.S., Weiner B.H., Dalen J.E. (1980). Unexplained chest pain in patients with normal coronary arteriograms. *The New England Journal of Medicine;* **303**:1249–1252.

Rose G. (1982). Incubation period of coronary heart disease. *British Medical Journal;* **284**:1600–1601.

Short D. (1976). Diseases of the cardiovascular system: treatment of angina. *British Medical Journal;* **2**:98–100.

Stubbe I., Eskilsson J., Nilsson-Ehle P. (1982). High-density lipoprotein concentrations increase after stopping smoking. *British Medical Journal;* **284**:1511–1513.

Thompson D.R. (1982). Ischaemic Heart Disease. In *Cardiac Nursing,* 1st edn., pp.133–205. London: Baillière Tindall.

Ward D.E., Camm A.J. (1981). Provocation of Arrhythmias. *Hospital Update;* **7**:391–402.

5

Myocardial Infarction

MYOCARDIAL INFARCTION

Myocardial infarction is defined as necrosis or death of cardiac muscle as the result of diminished oxygenated blood supply to the myocardium. Atherosclerosis causes progressive narrowing of the coronary areries and ultimately thrombosis leads to infarction. Occasionally, myocardial infarction can occur in patients who are later found to have normal coronary arteries. The mechanism here is presumed to be coronary artery spasm.

Physical signs

Myocardial infarction is characterised by severe and prolonged gripping retrosternal chest pain. The patient describes it as 'band-like' with radiation to the jaw and may even compare it with severe toothache. There may be radiation down the arms with a tingling sensation in the fingers. People who see the patient may describe his colour as ashen. The attack of pain may or may not have been preceded by angina pectoris and unlike that of angina pectoris, it is not relieved by rest or glyceryl trinitrate. Very occasionally, no history of chest pain is given.

During the early stages of infarction, the patient may have symptoms of nausea and vomiting. He may be cold and clammy and complain of shortness of breath. Generally, his condition will improve once his pain has been controlled. Sometimes there is a transient drop in blood pressure following myocardial infarction. This usually corrects itself as the patient's condition improves — unless the hypotension is associated with shock. Sometimes hypotension may be induced by analgesia.

Conversely, the patient may be hypertensive on arrival in the CCU. This hypertension may be transient and associated with pain and anxiety; it will often be rectified by relief of pain.

Diagnosis of Myocardial Infarction

A diagnosis of myocardial infarction can be made if two of the following criteria are fulfilled.
1. A well-defined history including prolonged chest pain.
2. ECG changes characteristic of transmural or subendocardial infarction.
3. A rise in serum enzymes.

Subendocardial infarction

This is an infarction which is limited to the muscle below the endocardium and it appears on the ECG as ST segment and T wave changes. Since these changes may reflect myocardial ischaemia, diagnosis of subendocardial infarction may be difficult but is confirmed by serum enzyme rise.

Transmural infarction

This is the term given to full thickness infarction which extends from the endocardium to the epicardium.

The Electrocardiograph in Myocardial Infarction

The evolution of myocardial infarction can be roughly divided into three stages. The first stage or acute stage is manifested on ECG by elevation of the ST segment in the leads over the injured area. It is coved in appearance extending into the T wave. The ST changes can occur within minutes of the onset of the infarction. ST depression may be seen in leads orientated towards the uninjured area of the heart; these may be reciprocal or mirror image changes, or may represent ischaemia (Fig. 5.1). The ST segment will return to normal within two or three days. Persistent

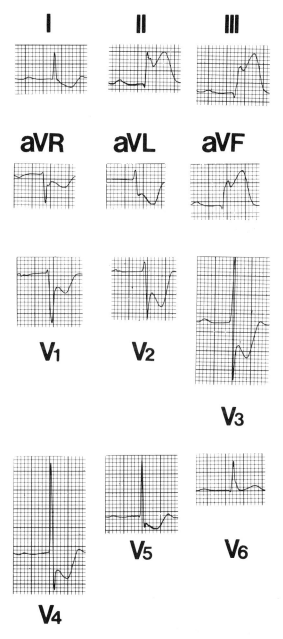

Fig. 5.1   An acute inferior myocardial infarction with anterior reciprocal changes and first degree block — PR interval of 0.32 seconds.

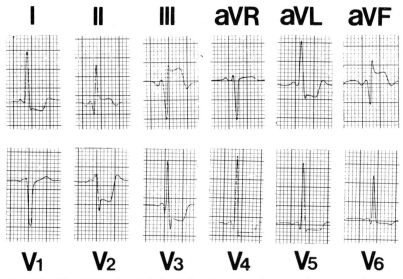

I   II   III   aVR   aVL   aVF

V1   V2   V3   V4   V5   V6

Fig. 5.2   The ECG of an inferior infarction showing development of Q waves and also anterior reciprocal changes. The rhythm is junctional.

ST elevation seen on the ECG months after infarction is suggestive of ventricular aneurysm.

The second stage of infarction on the ECG is the development of the pathological Q wave which is an indication of necrosis, cardiac muscle death (Fig. 5.2). The Q wave is present in the leads over the affected area and is wider than 0·04 seconds duration. It should be noted that a Q wave which will disappear with inspiration can be seen in standard lead III on the normal ECG. The Q wave reflects the absence of electrical activity in the infarction area. An electrode which is placed over the necrotic muscle of the left ventricle senses septal depolarisation (from left to right), and then depolarisation of both the right ventricle and left ventricle away from the injured zone. These negative forces summate to produce the deep pathological Q wave. This is also associated with loss of R wave amplitude. A full thickness infarction may result in a totally negative QS deflection in the leads over the necrosed area. The final stage is represented by T wave inversion, probably due to ischaemia. To summarise, the ST segment elevation signifies myocardial injury, while the development of the Q waves represents necrosis; T wave inversion is representative of myocardial ischaemia.

Myocardial Infarction Sites

Inferior Infarction

This is caused by diminished blood supply from the right or circumflex coronary artery (Fig. 2.11). The leads which demonstrate inferior infarction are leads II, III and aVF (Fig. 5.1 and Fig. 5.2). Sometimes additional lateral involvement is seen in V_4–V_6. The right coronary artery supplies the sino-atrial and atrioventricular nodes and inferior infarction is often associated with bradycardia and varying degrees of block (Fig. 5.1). Occasionally, branches of the right coronary artery which supply the right ventricle may be affected, resulting in right ventricular infarction. V_4, which is recorded on the right side of the chest, may assist in this diagnosis.

Posterior Infarction

As with inferior infarction, the site of occlusion may involve the right or circumflex coronary arteries (Fig. 2.11). This is demonstrated by tall R and T waves in leads V_1 and V_2 (Fig. 5.3) as these

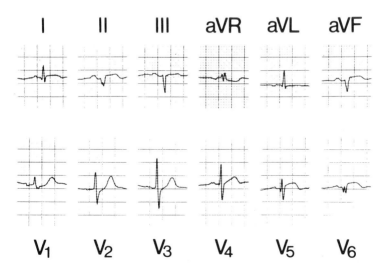

Fig. 5.3 *This ECG shows old inferior myocardial infarction and acute posterior infarction with lateral extension.*

are the leads opposite the site of necrosis. If the ECG is turned upside down and held up in front of a mirror, the reflection demonstrates the pathological Q wave and deep symmetrical T wave inversion typical of myocardial infarction (Fig. 5.4).

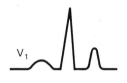

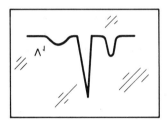

Fig. 5.4   Mirror image: if the ECG (top complex) is turned upside down and held up in front of a mirror, the reflection (bottom complex) shows the pathological Q wave and deep T wave inversion typical of myocardial infarction.

Anterior Infarction

This is due to the diminished blood supply of the left coronary artery (Fig. 2.12). The ECG shows extensive changes in leads I, aVL and V_1–V_6 (Fig. 5.5).

Anterolateral Infarction

The leads used to diagnose anterolateral infarction are leads I, aVL and V_4–V_6 (Fig. 5.6). It is the result of occlusion of the circumflex or diagonal branch of the left coronary artery.

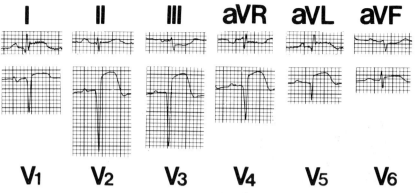

Fig. 5.5 An anterior myocardial infarction.

Anteroseptal Infarction

This is represented by changes in V_1 to V_4, as leads V_2 and V_3 lie directly over the septum which is supplied by the anterior descending branch of the left coronary artery (Fig. 5.7).

Difficult Localisation

Sometimes the site of infarction may be obscure and it may be necessary to record the ECG in the third intercostal space or using V_7 and V_8 to make diagnosis easier. An infarction occurring adjacent to previous myocardial necrosis may not produce clear new ECG changes.

Serum Enzymes

An enzyme is a protein which is formed in the cells and which changes the speed of chemical reactions. Serum enzymes are helpful in the diagnosis of myocardial infarction. If myocardial damage occurs enzymes are released into the blood stream, and can be measured. The enzymes which are released from damaged cardiac cells are:

1. creatine phosphokinase (CPK)
2. serum glutamic oxaloacetic transaminase (SGOT) or aspartate amino-transaminase (AST)
3. lactic dehydrogenase (LDH)

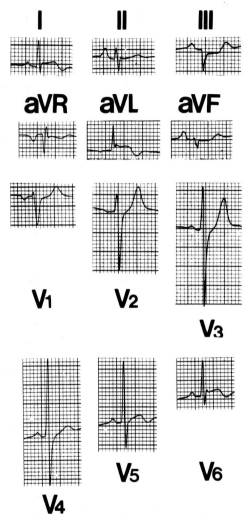

Fig. 5.6 An anterolateral myocardial infarction.

These enzymes are found in tissue other than the heart, for example, in the liver and skeletal muscle.

Serum Creatine Phosphokinase (CPK)

This is found in cardiac muscle, skeletal muscle and the brain. It is elevated following cardiopulmonary bypass or if the patient has

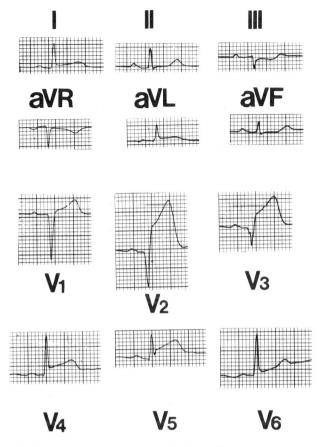

Fig. 5.7 An anteroseptal myocardial infarction.

been given an intramuscular injection. It rises within 6 hours of infarction and reaches its peak within 24 hours. The normal ranges in international units per litre (iu/litre) at 37° centigrade (C) are:

below 175 iu/litre for a male
below 140 iu/litre for a female

The CKMB isoenzyme is specific to cardiac muscle and is not influenced by intramuscular injections or musculoskeletal problems. At the present time, it is used in limited form only, because of expense. However, it is a valuable diagnostic aid to clarify the source of CPK elevation.

Serum Glutamic Oxaloacetic Transaminase (SGOT)

This enzyme rises within 12 hours following myocardial infarction, reaches its peak within 12–24 hours and remains elevated for three to five days. It is also found in the brain, liver and skeletal muscle. The normal range is below 37 iu/litre at 37°C.

Serum Lactic Dehydrogenase (LDH)

This is found in many tissues of the body, including the red cells and the heart. It reaches its peak 24–48 hours following the onset of myocardial infarction and remains elevated for up to three weeks. Because it is widely distributed, LDH is of limited use. However, it is often helpful in late diagnosis of myocardial infarction. The normal limits of LDH are 55–140 iu/litre at 25°C.

Figure 5.8 shows the different patterns of enzyme release after myocardial infarction. Hydroxybutyrate dehydrogenase (HBD) is another enzyme which some centres measure instead of LDH. Normal values of cardiac enzymes may vary from centre to centre as the result of different assay methods. Table 5.1 shows other conditions which may give elevated enzyme results.

Other Blood Tests

Blood samples are taken daily in the CCU for urea and electro-

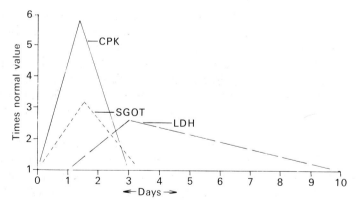

Fig. 5.8   Serum enzyme concentrations after myocardial infarction.

TABLE 5.1
Conditions other than myocardial infarction which may give
elevated serum enzyme concentrations.

CPK

DC Conversion	Vigorous muscular exercises
Stroke	Musculoskeletal disorders
Hypothyroidism	Cardiac catheterisation
Cardiopulmonary bypass sugery	

SGOT (AST)

Livcr discaso	Burns
Hypothyroidsim	Stroke
Administration of certain drugs	Muscle disease
Kidney, spleen, intestinal or pancreatic disorders	

LDH

Left ventricular failure
Liver, renal, muscle, blood or neoplastic disorders

lytes. Electrolyte imbalance (particularly imbalance of potassium and magnesium) may lead to cardiac arrhythmias. The ECG may help to make the diagnosis of electrolyte imbalance. The U wave is more dominant in hypokalaemia and the T wave becomes flattened and inverted. In hyperkalaemia the T wave becomes very tall and peaked and the QRS becomes widened. In very high potassium levels, the P wave eventually disappears.

A full blood count is taken on admission. A high white count and raised erythrocyte sedimentation rate (ESR) are normal reactions to myocardial necrosis. Later elevation of the ESR may help to diagnose Dressler's syndrome (post-myocardial infarction syndrome).

Blood is also taken on admission for blood glucose estimation. A transient initial rise is common, perhaps due to the stress of myocardial infarction. Alternatively, these patients may have diabetes which has not previously been diagnosed. Blood glucose often returns to normal quickly; however, patients showing a marked or persistent elevation may require further treatment.

NURSING AND MEDICAL MANAGEMENT OF PATIENTS FOLLOWING ACUTE MYOCARDIAL INFARCTION

Patients who have sustained acute myocardial infarction are admitted to CCUs for the prevention of complications or their early detection and treatment. These patients fall into one of three broad categories:

1. those who are admitted with no complications and who make an uncomplicated recovery.
2. those who are well on admission but who develop complications during their hospital stay.
3. those who are extremely ill on admission and whose progress depends primarily on the success of initial resuscitative measures.

The management of each patient is modified according to his individual needs.

Admission Priorities — the Patient

For the patient whose condition is stable, initial admission priorities include making him comfortable in bed and explaining what is happening. If every event is explained to the patient before it occurs, this will help to eliminate the fear and anxiety which accompanies loss of health and an uncertain future. Most patients are told that the chest pain they are experiencing may have been caused by a small heart attack and that they have been admitted to the CCU for relief of the pain and some simple investigations, the results of which will give more information about the heart attack. Although the event is not denied, the importance of it is minimised initially and the positive aspects are emphasised. Reference is frequently made to the many patients who return to a normal life-style after such an attack. Some patients can take in a lot of detail about their illness when they are first admitted. Others need time to get over the initial pain and shock before they can absorb the facts. However, no opportunity should be lost to emphasise that good progress is being made. The patient must also be encouraged to express how he is feeling about the situation. The 'listening' role of the nurse is fundamental to good practice.

Other admission priorities include commencing cardiac monitoring as soon as possible, as life threatening arrhythmias are common in the first few hours after myocardial infarction. A 12 lead ECG is recorded and measurements of blood pressure, temperature, heart rate and respiration rate are documented. Oxygen therapy may be commenced.

The doctor will examine the patient, insert an intravenous cannula and prescribe analgesia. He will also take blood samples and request a chest x-ray. The team of staff involved in the patient's care discuss his condition. They establish a plan of care and explain it to him, emphasising the importance of rest in bed and the reporting of further chest pain.

Admission Priorities — the Extremely Ill Patient

When a patient is in acute distress on admission, the priorities are different. The doctor must be contacted immediately. Emergency treatment may be required. Subsequent care depends on the severity of the patient's condition.

Admission Priorities — the Relatives

The calm, confident and friendly approach of the CCU staff is very reassuring for the patient and his relatives. Everyone reacts differently to admission to hospital and the relatives may be as anxious as the patient. They need time to talk and express their fears. They also require information about the patient's condition and plan of care. They should be taken to a quiet room where it can be explained to them in private that the patient may have had a heart attack. Individuals vary as to how much detail they can take in. The nurse must assess the situation and try to give the right amount of information at a suitable level for the person to whom she is talking. Many relatives want to know what a heart attack is. The nurse may describe it as a small area of heart muscle which has become damaged due to diminished blood supply. The relatives need to know about the investigations which will be performed and that they will be kept informed of the results. Some optimism is often expressed about the patient's prognosis if his condition is stable, but it is wise to warn relatives (and many are already aware) about the unpredictable nature of myocardial infarctions. Mention must also be made of the average length of stay in the CCU and the convalescent ward. Many relatives have questions they want to ask and they must be encouraged to do this both initially and each time they visit.

Details of the CCU visiting times and telephone number are given on a printed sheet, as these are easily forgotten in a stressful situation. Telephone communication is encouraged. This is often a main line of contact with the patient in units and wards where visiting is restricted to short periods.

Medical staff are always available to speak to the relatives and give further information about the patient's treatment and progress. The hospital chaplain is also pleased to give spiritual comfort to those who wish it. CCU staff must never forget that although the admission of a patient may be a routine event for them, it is a new, major and very frightening experience for the family involved. For the relatives of the patient who has sustained a massive myocardial infarction, the severity of the situation must be emphasised. Expressions like 'we are really very worried about Mr. Smith', certainly convey that the patients's condition is serious. However, it is often the tone of the nurse's voice and the expression on her face which communicate more than the words themselves. The nurse must observe the relatives' reaction closely — here too it is often non-verbal forms of communication which reveal how they are feeling. Sometimes they may derive comfort from the touch of a hand or an arm round their shoulders, but each situation is different and must be assessed individually.

Subsequent care

Following admission to the CCU, the condition of the patient who has suffered a myocardial infarction can change very quickly and the nurse must be constantly on the alert for this.

Bed Rest

Rest in bed is recommended for approximately 48 hours after admission, to encourage the recovery of the injured and ischaemic myocardium.

Analgesia

The patient must have adequate analgesia, usually intravenous morphine 10 mg or diamorphine 5 mg with an anti-emetic such as prochlorperazine 12·5 mg or metoclopramide 10 mg. The frequency of analgesia administration will depend on the response of the patient.

Observations

During his stay in the CCU, the patient's heart rhythm will be monitored continuously to detect dangerous arrhythmias. ECGs are recorded daily and if the diagnosis is in doubt, during and after pain.

The frequency of recordings of temperature, heart and respiratory rate and blood pressure will depend on the clinical status of the patient. However, they must be recorded regularly and changes reported. Pyrexia is common after myocardial infarction. Fluid intake and output must be recorded accurately, as diminished urine production may indicate possible renal damage due to hypotension following myocardial infarction.

Hygiene

For any patient in bed, meticulous hygiene is necessary, including a daily bed bath and regular care to pressure areas, mouth and hair.

Diet

Following myocardial infarction, the patient is often nauseated and anorexic. Special diets are unlikely to be tolerated initially; reducing diets for the obese are usually introduced at a later stage when the need to lose weight can be discussed rationally. Other patients such as diabetics, require a special diet from the time of admission. This can be organised easily with the help of the dietician, who is also involved in the follow-up care of many patients.

Elimination

The use of the commode is generally permitted, as it is thought to be less strenuous than balancing on a bedpan. Aperients are often necessary. Constipation should not be allowed to occur as it may induce straining. Suppositories are not now regarded as being contraindicated after myocardial infarction. Male patients may be allowed to stand out of bed to pass urine.

Physiotherapy

Physiotherapy is often commenced on the first day in hospital to prevent the complications of bed rest and to begin physical rehabilitation. This involves both nurses and trained physiotherapists and includes passive moments of the limbs and deep breathing exercises. The exercises become more vigorous during the convalescent period.

Intravenous Cannulae

All patients who have sustained an acute myocardial infarction have an intravenous cannula in place in case drugs are required quickly. These cannulae are checked regularly for evidence of bleeding, infection or thrombophlebitis. If displacement occurs, resiting will be necessary by the doctor. Cannulae which do not have a continuous intravenous infusion running through them are flushed regularly with heparin to maintain their patency. Dressings to cannulae are renewed if they are soiled or uncomfortable.

Anticoagulation

With current trends of early mobilisation after myocardial infarction, patients are not usually anticoagulated routinely unless they have specific risk factors for thrombus formation.

Medication

Medication after myocardial infarction is given as prescribed by the medical staff and patients are carefully observed for beneficial or adverse effects.

Social and Psychological Aspects

Home and work difficulties and other psychological problems of the patient must not be forgotten, even in the acute stages of myocardial infarction (see Chapter 9). The patient's level of anxiety must be assessed and the reasons for his excessive worry sought. Much reassurance can be derived from calm and caring staff who allow the patient to express his fears. Social problems causing anxiety may have adverse effects on the patient's general condition and may be best dealt with by the unit social worker.

Smoking

Smoking is not allowed in CCUs and patients are strongly advised to stop smoking altogether. Many are motivated to do this by the fear of having had a 'heart attack'. Others find that not being permitted to smoke adds to the anxiety of the situation. There is no easy answer; time must be spent with the patient to reinforce the dangers of continuing to smoke.

Transfer from the CCU

For the patient whose progress is uncomplicated in the CCU, transfer to a ward will occur approximately 48 hours after admission. Here complete physical and psychological rehabilitation will take place prior to discharge, between seven and ten days later. If the patient's progress on the CCU has been complicated, transfer may be delayed. Rehabilitation will have already begun in the CCU, but transfer out of the intensive area is a big psychological step. Apprehension is common and support from nursing staff is extremely important for the patient and his relatives.

It would be ideal if, before transfer from the CCU occurred, the patient and his closest relative could be seen together by a doctor and nurse. Their questions could be answered and the main aims of the convalescent period could be explained at this time. The patient may be anxious about getting on his feet, about being without his cardiac monitor and about the less close supervision that occurs on the follow-up ward. If he understands that he is making good progress, that such close observation is no longer necessary and that transfer out of the CCU is the first big step towards discharge, this may help to allay his anxiety. It would also be ideal for the patient and his relative to meet some of the convalescent ward staff, before the transfer is carried out. They would then feel less strange and isolated in the new surroundings. Ideally too, the relatives should be shown the ward to which the patient will be transferred. This is often a ward close to the CCU.

Unfortunately on busy CCUs, these 'ideals' are not always

possible and a compromise may have to be reached. The patient may have to be transferred before anticipated to vacate a bed for someone else. However, a patient should never be transferred without some time being spent with him to explain what is happening regarding his future care.

Convalescence — Physical, Social and Psychological Adaptations

The convalescent period calls for continued assessment of the patient's clinical condition in addition to observation of his social and psychological progress. Physical activity is gradually increased and the patient should be fully mobile and able to climb a flight of stairs prior to discharge from hospital. The patients often enjoy the social exchange with the other patients in the ward. They discuss mutual problems and may derive support from each other. However, the prospect of discharge may be very frightening.

Nursing priorities should aim to help the patient to achieve a suitable stage of physical, social and psychological independence to return to life at home. Re-education about life-style may be necessary. Community services may have to be organised. Information about medication, exercise, out-patient appointments and what to do if problems arise will certainly be required. Advice about driving will be necessary for many patients; driving can usually be resumed after a month. Patients who wish to fly should seek the advice of their doctor and the airline company but it is usually permissible between six and eight weeks after myocardial infarction.

Discussion about the resumption of sexual activity may embarrass patients and staff, and this advice is sometimes neither sought nor given. Patients should be reassured that normal sexual activity can be resumed after approximately one month provided they are progressing satisfactorily. If problems are encountered during sexual intercourse, they should be advised to speak to their family doctor. Sometimes patients may complain of impotence. This may be related to anxiety or drug therapy. Sympathetic counselling may be required or the drug prescription reviewed.

Information booklets are available and may be of help but these cannot replace advice from a member of staff. Many patients now have an exercise test before discharge and if no symptoms are encountered, they often find it very reassuring.

COMPLICATIONS OF MYOCARDIAL INFARCTION

Arrhythmias

Arrhythmias of varying degrees of severity are very common after myocardial infarction. These are discussed in detail in Chapter 6.

Left Ventricular Failure

Left ventricular failure (LVF) is the situation which arises when the left ventricle can no longer pump out sufficient blood for the needs of the body. When the left ventricle is damaged due to infarction, LVF is common.

The clinical feaures of LVF are mainly the result of diminished emptying of the left ventricle leading to increased pressure in the left atrium, pulmonary veins and capillaries. The signs and symptoms include dyspnoea, tachycardia, a third heart sound, pulmonary crepitations, pulmonary oedema and the production of frothy sputum which is sometimes tinged with blood. Anxiety often accompanies LVF. The treatment includes bed rest, oxygen, diuretics, the administration of diamorphine and an anti-emetic, and close observation of vital signs and urinary output.

Right Ventricular Failure

LVF may persist and progressive lung congestion will make it increasingly difficult for the right side of the heart to pump normally. The manifestations of right heart failure include raised jugular venous pressure, peripheral oedema and liver congestion as a result of the increasing backward pressure. Occasionally pleural effusion may occur. Right ventricular failure may also be a consequence of right ventricular infarction.

Cardiogenic Shock

Cardiogenic shock is a very serious complication of myocardial infarction. It suggests severe myocardial damage and results in decreased cardiac output with increased back pressure to the lungs. The fall in arterial blood pressure brings compensatory mechanisms into action, causing tachycardia and peripheral vasoconstriction. The signs and symptoms which result are those of poor perfusion of the tissues of the body. They include:

1. narrowing of the pulse pressure and hypotension.
2. coolness, pallor and sometimes clamminess of the peripheries of the body.
3. cerebral changes such as apathy, lethargy, confusion, disorientation and even coma.
4. diminishing urine output.
5. metabolic acidosis due to continuing metabolism without adequate oxygen supply (anaerobic metabolism).

Cardiogenic shock in the presence of extensive myocardial damage has a very poor prognosis.

The treatment is bed rest, oxygen, correction of acidosis, analgesia, diuretics and positive inotropic drugs to improve cardiac output and tissue perfusion. Careful observation of heart rate, blood pressure, respiration rate, intake and output is necessary.

Use of an arterial line will provide accurate measurements of arterial pressure and can be helpful for taking arterial blood samples for blood gas estimation. Normal blood gas estimations are shown in Table 5.2.

Urine output should be measured accurately with a urine catheter and urimeter. Central venous pressure and pulmonary artery capillary wedge pressure can be measured using a pulmonary artery catheter. This gives useful information about the severity of pulmonary congestion and circulatory fluid volume, in addition to assessing the effect of therapy. Mechanical cardiac assistance using the intra aortic balloon pump has only very limited value in this situation (see Chapter 11).

TABLE 5.2
Normal adult arterial blood gas estimations

pH	7.38 – 7.46
P_{CO_2}	4.26 – 6.12 kPa
P_{O_2}	9.84 – 14.36 kPa
HCO_3	21 – 29 mmol/litre
Base Excess	−2 – +2 mmol/litre
Oxygen Saturation	92 – 96%

Serious arrhythmias are often the terminal outcome of cardiogenic shock. The clinical features of cardiogenic shock may also be produced by hypovolaemia and slow heart rate and in these instances treatment is easier and the prognosis better.

Cardiac Rupture

Cardiac rupture is another serious complication of myocardial infarction. It may present as either rupture of the free ventricular wall or development of a ventricular septal defect.

Cardiac rupture is usually the result of extensive myocardial damage. The soft necrotic tissue weakens and eventually perforates. When it occurs as a rupture of the free ventricular wall, the blood flows out into the pericardial sac. This may produce cardiac tamponade and the heart becomes constricted by the build up of blood around it. Death usually follows quickly and attempts at resuscitation are rarely successful.

Rupture of the ventricular septum is also serious , but more can be done to treat it and improve tissue perfusion until surgery can be performed. The use of the intra aortic balloon pump has proved to be valuable in this situation. The main features of ventricular septal defect are usually chest pain and right ventricular failure, due to excessive left to right shunting of blood. A new systolic murmur is often heard at the left sternal edge. Atrioventricular or intraventricular conduction defects may appear on the electrocardiograph.

Papillary Muscle Dysfunction

Papillary muscle dysfunction occurs relatively commonly after myocardial infarction. It often produces some degree of malfunction of the chordae tendineae and thus mitral valve incompetence. The clinical features are usually those of LVF and the systolic murmur of mitral regurgitation will be audible.

Papillary Muscle Rupture

Papillary muscle rupture may sometimes complicate myocardial infarction. It is a serious situation giving rise to mitral valve incompetence, signs of severe LVF and a loud murmur throughout systole.

Pericarditis

Pericarditis is common two or three days after myocardial infarction. It results from irritation of the pericardium over the necrotic tissue. The signs and symptoms include chest pain which may mimic the pain of myocardial infarction, but which is usually worse on inspiration and movement and may be exacerbated by lying flat. It is usually associated with a pyrexia. A pericardial friction rub is often heard on ascultation. Electrocardiographic changes of acute pericarditis may show ST elevation with a concave upwards ST segment and peaked T waves (Fig. 5.9). These changes may be difficult to see in the patient who has pericarditis secondary to myocardial infarction. Soluble aspirin is usually an effective analgesic but other anti-inflammatory agents may be used.

Dressler's Syndrome

Pericarditis may also occur as a later complication in the weeks or months following myocardial infarction. This is sometimes called post-myocardial infarction syndrome or Dressler's syndrome. The clinical features are similar to those of acute pericarditis and the ESR will usually be significantly raised. If the pericarditis does not settle with bed rest and simple analgesics, corticosteroid therapy may occasionally be required.

Ventricular Aneurysm

Ventricular aneurysm may occur in the weeks after infarction. It results in paradoxical movement of the infarcted area of muscle. It may give features of LVF and increases the risk of systemic emboli and serious dysrhythmias.

Emboli

Both pulmonary and systemic emboli may follow infarction. Pulmonary emboli may cause chest pain, right heart failure, haemoptysis, cyanosis, tachycardia, hypotension and sweating (see Chapter 13). Characteristic ECG changes may be seen (Fig. 5.10). Pulmonary embolism was more common before the days of early mobilisation after myocardial infarction. The treatment

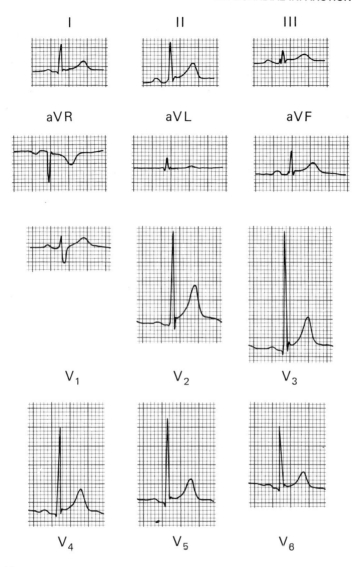

Fig. 5.9   The ECG of a patient with acute pericarditis.

includes analgesia, oxygen and anticoagulation.

Systemic emboli may also occur and result in transient cerebral ischaemia or stroke. Embolism to any peripheral artery may occur and despite the risk of anaesthesia after myocardial infarction, surgical embolectomy may have to be considered.

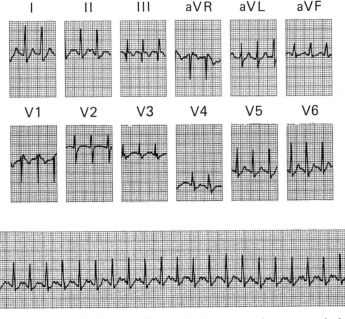

Fig. 5.10 The ECG of a patient with an acute pulmonary embolus showing an S wave in lead I, a Q wave, and an inverted T wave in lead III, and partial right bundle branch block.

Further Myocardial Infarction

Extension of existing myocardial infarction may also occur shortly after the initial event and the patient may remain at risk of further infarction in the future.

PROGNOSIS

The risk of death is greatest in the first few minutes after myocardial infarction. Awareness of this fact has stimulated considerable interest in the early admission of patients to specialised units. In some centres, casualty departments are bypassed and patients are brought directly to the CCU for assessment. Mobile coronary care units are used in some areas in an attempt to get treatment to the patient more quickly. Regrettably, despite these efforts, patients still die in the early hours after infarction. After 48 hours, mortality decreases significantly. This may allow patients who are seen for the first time more than 48 hours after infarction to be cared for at home, if the infarction is uncomplicated and the social circumstances are favourable. Hypertension, angina or previous myocardial infarction, old age, extensive infarction or complications such as prolonged pain, LVF, cardiogenic shock or arrhythmias, suggest a less favourable prognosis.

Further Reading

Andreoli K.G., Hunn-Fowkes V., Zipes D.P., Wallace A.G. (1979), *Comprehensive Cardiac Care: a Text for Nurses, Physicians and Other Health Practitioners*, 4th edn. St. Louis: The C.V. Mosby Company.

Ashworth P. (1981). Communicating with Patients and Relatives in the Intensive Care Unit. In *Communication in Nursing Care* (Bridge W., Clark J.M., eds.) pp. 64–82. London: HM and M Publishers.

Ashworth P. (1984). Communicating in an intensive care unit. In *Communication* (Faulkner A., ed.) pp.94–112. Edinburgh: Churchill Livingstone.

Cay E.L. (1982). Psychological Aspects of Cardiac Rehabilitation. *Hospital Update;* 8:161–170.

Hampton J.R. (1978). Coronary care: the management of suspected myocardial infarction. *British Journal of Hospital Medicine;* 20:242–246.

Julian D.G. (1983). Disease of the Coronary Arteries. In *Cardiology*, 4th edn., pp.125–162. London: Baillière Tindall.

Julian D.G., Matthews M.B. (1977). Diseases of the Cardiovascular System. In *Davidson's Principles and Practice of Medicine: a Textbook for Students and Doctors*. (Macleod J., ed.) 12th edn., pp.171–247. Edinburgh: Churchill Livingstone.

Malcolm A.D. (1980). Anticoagulants for heart disease. *British Journal of Hospital Medicine;* 23:606–615.

McLeod A.A., Jewitt D.E. (1978). Role of 24 hour ambulatory electrocardiographic monitoring in a general hospital. *British Medical Journal;* 1:1197–1199.

Meltzer L.E., Dunning A.J., eds. (1972). *Textbook of Coronary Care.* Amsterdam: Excerpta Medica.

Meltzer L.E., Pinneo R., Kitchell J.R. (1977). Acute Myocardial Infarction; Coronary Care Nursing; The Major Complications of Acute Myocardial Infarction and the Related Nursing Role. In *Intensive Coronary Care: a manual for nurses*, 3rd edn., pp.13–22; 57–74; 75–108. Bowie, Md.: The Charles Press Publishers.

Norris R.M. (1982). *Myocardial Infarction.* Edinburgh: Churchill Livingstone.

Portal R.W. (1982). Elective surgery after myocardial infarction. *British Medical Journal;* **284**:843–844.

Resnekov L. (1978). Coronary Care: Cardiogenic Shock. *British Journal of Hospital Medicine;* **20**:232–241.

Schamroth L. (1977). *An introduction to electrocardiography.* Oxford: Blackwell.

Schamroth L. (1972). The electrocardiographic diagnosis of acute myocardial infarction. In *Textbook of Coronary Care* (Meltzer L.E., Dunning A.J., eds.). pp.61–81. Amsterdam: Excerpta Medica.

Sime A.M. (1983). Lessening patient stress in the CCU. *Nursing Management;* **14** (**10**):24–26.

Singer D.E., Mulley A.G., Thibault G.E., Barnett G.O. (1981). Unexpected Re-admissions to the Coronary Care Unit during recovery from acute myocardial infarction. *The New England Journal of Medicine;* **304**:625–629.

Thompson D.R. (1982). Ischaemic Heart Disease. In *Cardiac Nursing,* 1st edn., pp.133–205. London: Baillière Tindall.

Toth J.C. (1980). Effect of structured preparation for transfer on patient anxiety, on leaving coronary care unit. *Nursing Research;* **29** (**1**): 28–34.

Wilson-Barnett J. (1984). Coping with Stress. *Nursing Mirror;* **158** (**14**):16.

Zannetton M. (1981). Intensive therapy: patients are people. *Nursing Mirror;* **150** (**3**): 27.

6

Cardiac Arrhythmias

An arrhythmia may be described as any cardiac rhythm which deviates from normal sinus rhythm (Fig. 6.1). It may be regular or irregular. An ectopic rhythm is an arrhythmia originating from other than the sinus node. An extrasystole is a premature beat interupting the normal regular rhythm. An escape ectopic beat terminates a pause in the regular rhythm and is not premature (Fig. 6.2). It is important to differentiate between these since extrasystoles may require drug suppression whereas escape beats are considered as safety mechanisms.

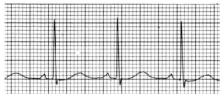

Fig. 6.1   Sinus rhythm.

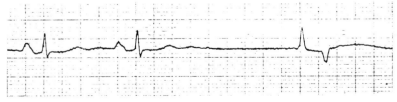

Fig. 6.2   A junctional escape beat.

There are two important mechanisms by which ectopic beats and arrhythmias may develop:

1. Enhanced Automaticity

During diastole, all the cells in the conducting system undergo spontaneous depolarisation. This is a characteristic property of all potential pacemaker cells and differentiates them from myocardial muscle cells. When the transmembrane potential falls to a certain level, referred to as the threshold, an impulse is formed and conducted. Whichever cell reaches threshold first will therefore initiate the heart beat. Usually the sinus node depolarises quickest and controls the heart rhythm. If, however, another cell elsewhere spontaneously depolarises faster than the sinus node, then it will reach threshold first and produce an ectopic beat. Since depolarisation of all pacemaker cells occurs automatically, when it occurs faster than normal it is referred to as enhanced automaticity (Fig. 6.3).

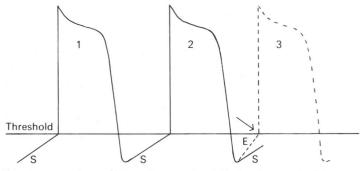

Action potentials 1 and 2 are initiated by the sinus node (S). Action potential 3 represents an extrasystole due to an ectopic focus depolarising quicker, to reach threshold (arrow) (E) before the sinus node.

Fig. 6.3   Enhanced automaticity.

2. Re-entry

Although a nerve can be conveniently considered as a single pathway for electrical stimulation, in reality it is composed of many individual fibres bundled together rather like an electrical cable. In the heart, this arrangement allows the opportunity for disordered conduction to produce extrasystoles and arrhythmias.

This concept can be simplified by imagining two conducting fibres, A and B, joined at the top and bottom but insulated from

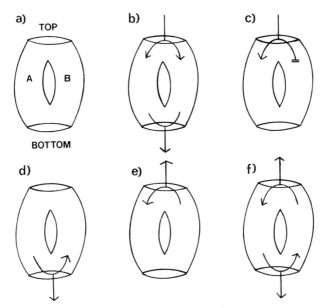

Fig. 6.4 Diagram to show the re-entry mechanism.

each other in the middle (Fig. 6.4a). Normally, an impulse travelling downwards will pass through both fibres and converge at the bottom (Fig. 6.4b). If the impulse enters early at the top and finds B refractory, it will conduct downwards only through A (Fig. 6.4c). When it reaches the bottom, B will have recovered and the impulse can travel backwards along this fibre (Fig. 6.4d). It can be considered as having re-entered the conducting tissue. When it reaches the top of B, A may have recovered and may allow it to travel downwards again (Fig. 6.4e). Thus a self-perpetuating re-entry circuit may be established (Fig. 6.4f).

The anatomy of the AV node and the widespread ramifications of the Purkinje network are ideally structured to permit re-entry. It is of clinical importance since a single extrasystole may provoke a sustained tachycardia. It is often much easier to prevent the arrhythmia by giving a drug that blocks the re-entry circuit rather than attempting to totally eradicate all the extrasystoles that might initiate the mechanism.

Arrhythmias are often associated with cardiac disease, but they may occur in otherwise normal healthy people who have no history of cardiac or any other abnormality. Arrhythmias are also a complication of endocrine disorders such as thyrotoxicosis and may be seen as a result of pulmonary embolism or infarction, hypothermia, drug administration and electrolyte imbalance.

DISORDERS OF SINUS RHYTHM

Sinus Tachycardia

This is the term used to describe a rhythm with a rate of more than 100 beats per minute. The origin is in the SA node and it produces the normal P waves and QRST complexes on the ECG recording. It is a normal response to emotion and to exercise. It is sometimes caused by drugs such as atropine or adrenaline. Sinus tachycardia may be present in myocardial infarction, but it may also be associated with cardiac failure, thyrotoxicosis and fever.

Sinus Bradycardia

Sinus bradycardia is defined as a heart rate of less than 60 beats per minute originating in the SA node (Fig. 6.5). It is not associated with any change in the P or QRST complexes. It is common in patients receiving beta adrenoreceptor blocking agents. It may be

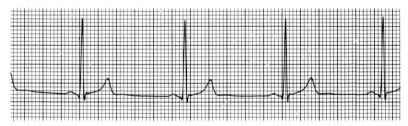

Fig. 6.5   Sinus bradycardia.

found in athletes but it also results from the vagal response evoked by fear or pain. Patients with inferior myocardial infarction commonly suffer episodes of sinus bradycardia. No treatment is required unless it is associated with symptoms, in which case atropine may be given.

Sinus Arrhythmia

Sinus arrhythmia is characterised by phasic changes in the heart

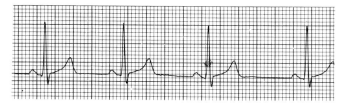

Fig. 6.6   Sinus arrhythmia.

rate associated with respiration (Fig. 6.6). The faster rate is associated with inspiration and the slower rate with expiration. The P wave and QRST complex are normal. No treatment is required.

Sinus Arrest

Sinus arrest describes the absence of a complete PQRS complex. The sinus node is depressed and fails to generate an impulse; a pacemaker situated in the AV junction takes over and a junctional escape rhythm results. If sinus arrest causes a symptomatic fall in the cardiac output, atropine may be given intravenously to lessen the vagal overactivity.

In sino-atrial block, the impulses may originate normally but are blocked within the node and subsequently fail to reach the atria; this results in a complete absence of a PQRST complex (Fig. 6.7). (See Chapter 7 — Conduction Defects.)

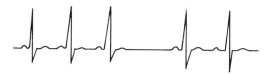

Fig. 6.7   Sino-atrial block with one omitted PQRST complex.

SUPRAVENTRICULAR ARRHYTHMIAS

These are arrhythmias which originate above the ventricles and can be divided into atrial and junctional.

Atrial Ectopic Beats

Atrial ectopic beats are benign single early beats and are often

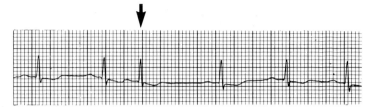

Fig. 6.8 *Atrial ectopic (indicated by arrow).*

found in the normal healthy individual (Fig. 6.8). An increase in frequency may be a forewarning of a more serious arrhythmia. The impulse arises from an ectopic focus in the atria resulting in an abnormal P wave. Usually the QRST complex is narrow and similar to that of the patient's complex when in sinus rhythm. The P wave may be obscured and is often difficult to see on a monitor lead; lead V_1 on the ECG is usually the best lead for identifying the P wave. A compensatory pause follows the ectopic beat. If one atrial ectopic beat follows a sinus beat on a regular basis, this is termed atrial bigeminy.

Atrial Fibrillation

This is the most common potentially serious atrial arrhythmia (Fig. 6.9). It is described as ectopic atrial activity of greater than 300 beats per minute and because of the very fast rate, no definite P waves are seen on the ECG. The bizarre and irregular baseline is due to disorganised and chaotic atrial depolarisation. There is always some degree of block at the AV node, since it cannot conduct beats at this fast rate and therefore only some of the impulses reach the ventricles. The QRST complex is narrow and is similar to that of the patient in sinus rhythm, but here the RR interval is irregular.

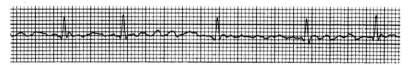

Fig. 6.9 *Atrial fibrillation.*

Nurses should record both the apex rate and pulse rate in patients with atrial fibrillation. The apex rate is usually faster than the radial beat, because some beats are so weak that they cannot be felt at the radial pulse.

Depending upon the ventricular rate, which is often 120–160 beats per minute but may be faster or slower, treatment may or may not be initiated. Atrial fibrillation may be found in the patient with myocardial infarction and is frequently associated with cardiac failure. It may also relate to pulmonary embolus and mitral valve disease. Atrial fibrillation can occur in patients with thyrotoxicosis and constrictive pericarditis, while paroxysmal atrial fibrillation is seen in some patients with the Wolff–Parkinson–White syndrome. Treatment may depend on whether the event is new or longstanding. Nothing may be gained by trying to restore sinus rhythm when the arrhythmia has been known to exist long-term and has not caused complications.

In patients with myocardial infarction, atrial fibrillation may be transient. However, fast fibrillation may cause haemodynamic complications and it may, therefore, be necessary to cardiovert using DC shock followed by anti-arrhythmic therapy. Where the need to restore sinus rhythm is not so urgent, the patient may be digitalised. In some cases, it may be necessary to add a beta blocker to slow the ventricular rate for patients in whom the arrhythmia is proving to be resistant to digitalis therapy. Patients with mitral valve disease may require anticoagulants as they are at risk from systemic embolism.

Atrial Flutter

Atrial flutter may arise as the result of a re-entry mechanism and occurs at a rate of 250–300 beats per minute (Fig. 6.10). Usually there is 2:1 or 3:1 AV block; if the rate is 300, the ventricular rate in 2:1 block would therefore be 150 per minute. There is no normal P wave to be seen, but flutter waves generally give a saw-toothed appearance, which can be best revealed when the block is increased by carotid sinus massage (Fig. 6.11). The QRS complex is unchanged. Atrial flutter may be present in myocardial

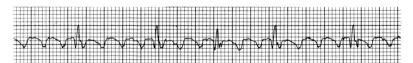

Fig. 6.10   Atrial flutter.

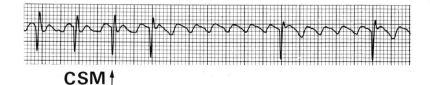

CSM↑

Fig. 6.11 Atrial flutter showing increased block by carotid sinus massage (CSM).

infarction, rheumatic heart disease or thyrotoxicosis. It may be transient, but may degenerate to atrial fibrillation and be a precursor of cardiac failure.

As with atrial fibrillation, it may be necessary to consider cardioversion. In non-urgent cases, digoxin may be used to increase AV block.

Supraventricular Tachycardia

In supraventricular tachycardia impulses occur from 150–250 beats per minute and rise in the atria or junctional tissue (Fig. 6.12). The QRS complex is usually unchanged, but the P wave may be obscured and may be buried in the QRS complex. Supraventricular tachycardia can be said to be present when three or more successive supraventricular ectopic beats are observed to occur at a fast rate. Carotid sinus massage may help in the diagnosis by terminating the arrhythmia and restoring sinus rhythm. Supraventricular tachycardia which reoccurs in bursts and disappears spontaneously is called paroxysmal supraventricular tachycardia. It is often encountered in otherwise healthy young people. In this context it is seldom dangerous and can usually be left to stop on its own; or it can be terminated by Valsalva manoeuvre or carotid sinus pressure. The electrocardiograph when the patient is in sinus rhythm is usually normal, but may give the appearance of Wolff–Parkinson–White or Lown–

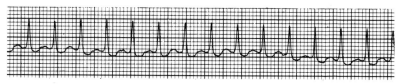

Fig. 6.12 Supraventricular tachycardia.

Ganong–Levine syndrome (short P–R syndrome). In myocardial infarction, however, it may quickly produce cardiac failure and hypotension. If hypotension is present, DC cardioversion is necessary; otherwise, drug therapy is administered.

There is a form of supraventricular tachycardia (atrial tachycardia with block) in which some of the impulses are blocked in their passage to the ventricles, for example, 2:1 block, with an atrial rate of 180 and a ventricular rate of 90. It is important to recognise this as it is frequently a consequence of digitalis toxicity associated with potassium depletion. In such circumstances digitalis is contraindicated and potassium should be administered.

Junctional (Nodal) Ectopic Beats

These are ectopic beats arising from the AV junction. The atria are depolarised retrogradely from the AV node resulting in inverted 'P' waves in II, III and AVF. The 'P' wave may precede, follow or be buried in the QRS complex.

Junctional Rhythm

Junctional rhythm results when the junctional area takes over as the pacemaker of the heart (Fig. 6.13). The heart rate is slower than normal, often under 60 beats per minute. On the ECG, the P wave may precede the QRS complex, follow it or it may be buried in the QRS complex. If the P wave is in front of the complex, the P–R interval will be short, that is less than 0·12 seconds.

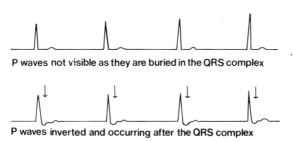

P waves not visible as they are buried in the QRS complex

P waves inverted and occurring after the QRS complex

Fig. 6.13   Junctional rhythm.

VENTRICULAR ARRHYTHMIAS

Ventricular arrhythmias result from abnormal electrical activity in the ventricles. They are often seen in patients who have sustained a myocardial infarction, but they may also be associated with cardiac failure, hypoxia, hypokalaemia and drugs and can be due to re-entry or enhanced automaticity.

Ventricular Ectopic Beats

These beats occur prematurely and are not preceded by a P wave (Fig. 6.14). The QRS complex is broad, unlike that in sinus rhythm, and is usually followed by a compensatory pause. When a ventricular ectopic follows each sinus beat, this is termed ventricular bigeminy (Fig. 6.15). The term ventricular trigeminy is used to describe a repeating pattern of two sinus beats followed by one ventricular ectopic beat (Fig. 6.16).

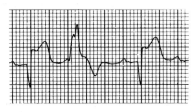

Fig. 6.14   An isolated ventricular ectopic occurring in a patient with acute myocardial infarction.

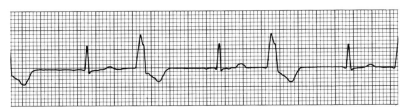

Fig. 6.15   One ventricular ectopic following each sinus beat, i.e. ventricular bigeminy.

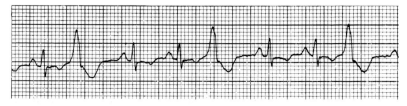

Fig. 6.16   Ventricular trigeminy.

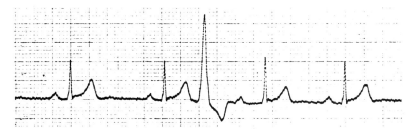

Fig. 6.17 An interpolated ectopic not interrupting the normal rhythm. However, the beat following the ectopic shows a long PR interval.

The term interpolated ectopic beat is used to describe a ventricular ectopic beat which is 'sandwiched' between two normal sinus beats and does not interrupt normal sinus rhythm (Fig. 6.17). If all ectopic beats are of the same configuration, they are called uniform; if of more than one type, they are termed multiform.

It has long been felt that ectopic beats of the R on T variety are liable to induce ventricular fibrillation in patients who have sustained a myocardial infarction. Frequent ventricular ectopic beats are treated in some hospitals, but research over the years has shown that conventional lignocaine therapy may be of no benefit. Some centres are less aggressive in treating ventricular ectopics. Ventricular ectopic beats have been seen on 24 hour tapes of normal individuals.

Ventricular Tachycardia

Ventricular tachycardia is the result of a rapidly discharging focus originating in the ventricles at a rate greater than 120 beats per minute (Fig. 6.18). On the ECG, the QRS complexes are seen to be broad and bizarre and the P waves may be dissociated or unidentifiable. When the tachycardia is prolonged, the patient becomes hypotensive and may develop left ventricular failure. The urgency of treatment depends on the haemodynamic state.

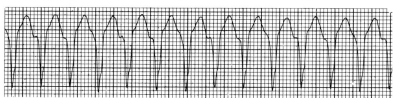

Fig. 6.18 Ventricular tachycardia.

Elective DC conversion may be required. If the patient becomes unconscious, then emergency defibrillation will be performed. Intravenous lignocaine 50–150 mg as a bolus is given over two to five minutes, followed by an infusion of lignocaine at 4 mg/minute and then 3 mg/minute for half an hour each in turn, followed by 2 mg/minute for 24 hours.

Patients who develop recurrent ventricular tachycardia, other than those who have sustained myocardial infarction, require full investigation including electrophysiology and angiography. Anti-arrhythmic therapy may then be prescribed or surgery may be suggested.

Accelerated Idioventricular Rhythm

This is in effect slow ventricular tachycardia (Fig. 6.19). The origin is again in the ventricles and the QRS complex is broad. However, the rate of 60–100 beats per minute is slower than that of ventricular tachycardia. It is transient and rarely requires treatment, unless accompanied by the faster ventricular tachycardia.

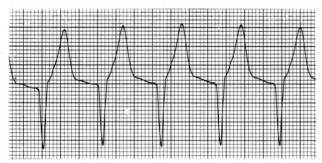

Fig. 6.19 Accelerated idioventricular rhythm.

Ventricular Fibrillation

Ventricular fibrillation is the most common cause of sudden death and is particularly associated with recent myocardial infarction (Fig. 6.20). However, it is not limited to this group of patients; it also occurs in patients with ischaemic heart disease without infarction, cardiomyopathies and many other disorders. In ventricular fibrillation, there is disorganised and rapid action of the heart without effective contraction. There is no coordination of

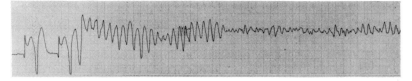

Fig. 6.20   Ventricular fibrillation.

the atria and ventricles and the rate will be from 300–500 beats per minute. Sometimes the complexes give a regular appearance and this is called ventricular flutter. If treatment of this arrhythmia is not instigated, the appearance of the fibrillation becomes finer and eventually terminates into asystole. Ventricular fibrillation may be described as 'primary' when it occurs in the early hours of myocardial infarction and is not associated with severe cardiac damage; primary ventricular fibrillation responds readily to treatment. 'Secondary' ventricular fibrillation implies severe impairment of the myocardium and is a result of shock or cardiac failure. 'Late' ventricular fibrillation occurs one to six weeks post-infarction. The prognosis is poor for secondary and late ventricular fibrillation because of the associated myocardial damage.

The treatment for ventricular fibrillation is DC electroconversion. The initial shock is 200 joules increasing to 400 joules if necessary. A lignocaine bolus of 50–150 mg is given with a lignocaine infusion as prescribed. Uncomplicated primary ventricular fibrillation needs no further treatment following the initial emergency treatment. Patients who have sustained secondary or late ventricular fibrillation may require further anti-arrhythmic treatment (see Chapter 16).

Torsade De Pointes

Torsades de Pointes is ventricular tachycardia characterised by 'twisting of the points' of the QRS complex, the appearance of the complexes changing every few beats. It is not uncommonly found in patients with a long Q–T interval; it may be associated with drug therapy or it may be congenital. It is usually self-terminating. Otherwise it may be abolished by pacing, by correcting electrolyte imbalance or by withdrawing the responsible drugs.

Dying Heart

This is very slow activity of the ventricles not associated with

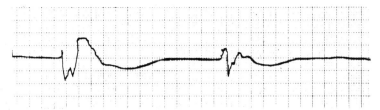

Fig. 6.21 A dying heart.

purposeful contractions; it is commonly seen at the end of resuscitative measures (Fig. 6.21). It is referred to as a dying heart pattern and indicates a terminal situation. Pacing is not effective.

CARDIAC ARREST

Cardiac arrest is the sudden cessation of the pumping of the heart and may be due to ventricular fibrillation or asystole. Treatment

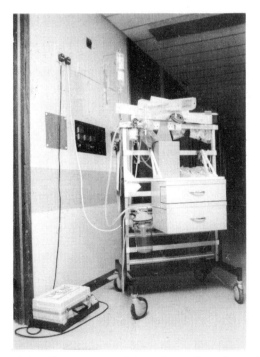

Fig. 6.22a A cardiac arrest trolley — front view. A small portable defibrillator can be seen on the left hand side.

must be initiated immediately, as prolonged cardiac arrest over four minutes invariably causes brain cell damage. In the CCU it is often the result of myocardial infarction or ischaemia; it may also be the result of drugs or electrolyte imbalance. Outside the hospital, cardiac arrest may be due to myocardial infarction or ischaemia, drug therapy, electrocution or unknown causes. In the coronary care unit, diagnosis can be made from the monitor, but outside the coronary care unit, diagnosis is made by the loss of arterial pulsation. It is essential that the femoral or carotid pulse is used as the radial may be impalpable for some other reason. Loss of consciousness follows. Respiration becomes stertorous and may cease; these signs are adequate for a diagnosis of cardiac arrest. Inspection of the pupils will show dilatation. The member of staff who finds the patient should summon help and while awaiting the emergency equipment (Fig. 6.22a and b); place the patient flat and remove the patient's dentures. He or she should give a swift, sharp blow over the sternum, as this action will occasionally

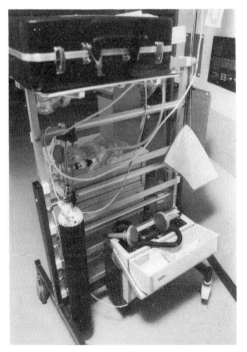

Fig. 6.22b The rear view of cardiac arrest trolley incorporating defibrillator.

restart the heart, and then commence external cardiac massage. Both hands are placed over the sternum enabling rhythmic compression to take place. It must be carried out firmly but not too forcefully, as fracture of the ribs may occur. An airway should be placed in the patient's mouth and if no breathing bag is available, mouth to mouth breathing must be employed. Once the emergency equipment has been obtained, an ambu bag with oxygen can be used to give ventilatory assistance. If the arrest is prolonged, an endotracheal tube may be used.

Acidosis may develop. This can be corrected by infusing 50–100 m/equivalents of 8·4% sodium bicarbonate. Arterial blood should be sampled to check on blood gases and pH. Normal arterial gases are shown in Table 5.2 in Chapter 5.

Emergency Defibrillation

If the cardiac arrest is caused by ventricular fibrillation, immediate DC conversion from 200–400 joules (watt/second) is necessary. Defibrillators are operated either from a battery or from the mains electricity supply. Battery operated defibrillators should always be left on charge when not in use.

The defibrillator is operated by trained personnel who appreciate the safety hazards. The operator may be a member of the medical staff or a member of the nursing staff who is legally permitted to defibrillate.

Electrode jelly or impregnated pads are placed on the right side of the upper chest and below the left axilla, protecting the patient's skin from burns. The defibrillator is switched on and charged to the selected energy. Before the shock is delivered, all staff move away from the bed while the operator places the paddles firmly on the chest and then depresses the switch on the paddles to deliver the charge. The shock depolarises the heart, thus abolishing all electrical activity temporarily. When the heart starts to function again, the sinus node should take over as primary pacemaker and re-establish sinus rhythm.

Following cardioversion, the patient should be given a bolus of lignocaine and an infusion of lignocaine should be commenced, as described previously. Oral anti-arrhythmic agents may be prescribed for patients with secondary fibrillation.

Electrical equipment in the coronary care unit should be regularly inspected for faults and any new apparatus should be checked by the electrical engineer. Locker surfaces and floor surfaces should be kept clean and dry in areas where defibrillators are required.

Cardiac Arrest due to Ventricular Asystole

Asystole is the term used to describe the absence of myocardial activity. The prognosis is very poor.

The immediate emergency measures of cardiac arrest with asystole include cardiac compression and assistance with ventilation. Sodium bicarbonate should be infused to correct acidosis. Isoprenaline, which increases both atrial and ventricular rates and improves myocardial contraction, may be given as a bolus of 100 µg; an infusion of isoprenaline may be used for maintenance. Calcium chloride may be given to increase myocardial tone. Adrenaline 1:10 000 in 10 mls may be given intravenously or by intracardiac injection. It should be noted that to prevent precipitation, any line used to give sodium bicarbonate should be flushed with sodium chloride before giving calcium. In cases of asystole, it may be necessary to insert a temporary pacing wire to establish a rhythm.

SYNCHRONISED DC CONVERSION

This is used to convert atrial and ventricular tachycardia electively. It is indicated for patients in whom the arrhythmia is not immediately life-threatening, but in whom it has caused haemodynamic impairment and cardiac failure. The patient should sign a written consent once the procedure has been explained. A general anaesthetic may be given; alternatively, intravenous valium can be used as sedation. The technique for defibrillation is the same as described earlier, but the level of energy selected is lower, such as 50 joules (watt/second). This may be increased if the initial lower energy selection fails. It is important to synchronise the timing of the shock to avoid the vulnerable period (the T wave) as ventricular fibrillation may occur. Generally speaking, it is advisable to avoid DC conversation if digitalis has been prescribed, as serious ventricular arrhythmias may be induced.

USE OF PACING WIRES IN TACHYARRHYTHMIAS

Artificial pacing can be used to control tachyarrhythmias. A quadripolar or hexipolar pacing wire is introduced to the right ventricle, and attached to a battery operated pacing box. It is usually necessary to pace at a higher rate than the tachycardia ('overdrive'). The pacemaker will capture the heart's rhythm and when the pacing is abruptly discontinued, sinus rhythm should be restored. Sometimes pacing at a lower rate ('underdrive') is effective in terminating the arrhythmia.

A conventional pacing apparatus usually does not allow pacing at sufficiently high rates for overdrive pacing; appropriately modified boxes are available (see Fig. 8.1).

Further Reading

Julian D.G. (1983). Disorders of Rate, Rhythm and Conduction. In *Cardiology*, 4th edn., pp.49–64. London: Baillière Tindall.

Meltzer L.E., Pinneo R., Mitchell J.R. (1977). *Intensive Coronary Care.* 3rd edn., Bowie, Md.: The Charles Press Publishers.

Norris R.M. (1982). *Myocardial Infarction.* Edinburgh: Churchill Livingstone.

Schamroth L. (1977). *An introduction to electrocardiography*, 5th edn. Oxford: Blackwell.

7

Conduction Defects

Conduction disturbances may arise in the SA node, the AV node and bundle of His (together called the AV junction), and the left and right bundle branches.

CONDUCTION DEFECTS ARISING IN THE SA NODE

SA Block

In SA block the impulse is formed normally in the SA node, but it fails to be conducted to the atria. On the monitor it is impossible to distinguish SA block from SA arrest in which no impulse is formed by the SA node. In SA block one or more PQRS complexes are omitted; when the next normal PQRS occurs, it will arrive on time (Fig. 7.1). However, a lower pacemaker may take over and produce an escape beat or rhythm.

The causes of SA block include degenerative fibrosis, ischaemia

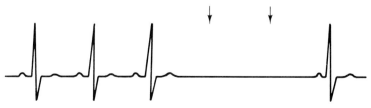

Fig. 7.1   Sino-atrial block showing two omitted PQRST complexes.

and excessive vagal influence to the SA node. Administration of certain drugs can block impulses within the SA node. Symptomatic SA block is a clinical feature of sick sinus syndrome.

Often no treatment is required. However, should the patient have a marked reduction in heart rate and suffer symptoms associated with diminished cardiac output, atropine therapy may be effective by removing vagal tone. If the arrhythmia is drug-induced, the drug should be discontinued. Very rarely temporary pacing may be required.

CONDUCTION DEFECTS ARISING IN THE AV JUNCTION

Conduction defects which occur in the AV junction are divided into first, second and third degree block. They may occur in or around the AV node or high or low in the bundle of His. There are many reasons for such blocks occurring: drugs (digoxin, beta-blockers, verapamil), metabolic disturbances, chronic fibrosis of the conducting pathways, ischaemia, myocardial infarction and viral disorders affecting the heart.

First Degree AV Block

In first degree AV block the impulse is formed normally in the SA node but its conduction between the atria and ventricles is delayed, resulting in a prolonged PR interval of over 0·20 seconds. The rhythm is regular and the heart rate is undisturbed (Fig. 7.2). It rarely produces any symptoms and is not often treated. The main danger associated with the arrhythmia is that it may proceed to more serious degrees of block.

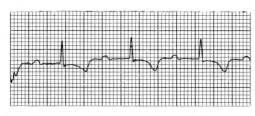

Fig. 7.2   First degree AV block — PR interval of approximately 0.28 seconds.

Second Degree AV Block

The second degree AV blocks are further sub-divided into:

1. Wenckebach phenomenon (Mobitz type 1).
2. Mobitz type II.

The second degree AV blocks are characterised by normal P waves, some of which are not conducted to the ventricles.

Wenckebach phenomenon

In Wenckebach phenomenon, the block usually occurs above the bundle of His, resulting in progressive delay in AV conduction until finally one impulse is not conducted. On the ECG monitor, there appears progressive lengthening of the PR interval for several complexes. Then, with the non-conducted impulse, a normal P wave appears but is not followed by a QRS complex. The cycle then begins again and repeats itself. Each cycle commonly has two, three, four or five conducted beats before the non-conducted one. The RR interval is greatest between the two beats following the non-conducted P, as the incremental delay in conduction time is greatest in the second beat of the cycle. The RR interval then decreases and before the next non-conducted P, should always be shorter than the RR interval following it (Fig. 7.3).

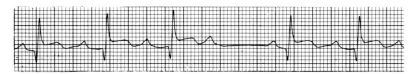

Fig. 7.3 Wenckebach phenomenon showing three conducted beats before the non-conducted P. Note that the RR interval is greatest between the two beats following the non-conducted P.

It is unusual for the patient with Wenckebach phenomenon to have symptoms which require treatment, as most beats are conducted to the ventricles. The main danger of this arrhythmia is that it may lead to more serious degrees of block, particularly when it occurs in association with acute myocardial infarction.

Mobitz type II

Mobitz type II may present with what appears to be normal sinus rhythm with occasional non-conducted P waves. More usually the block is regular; for example, in 2:1 AV block, the ECG monitor picture will repeatedly show one P wave conducted to the ventricles followed by one which is not conducted. The PR interval is always constant and may be within normal limits of duration (Fig. 7.4) or prolonged. In 3:1 AV block, only every third P wave is conducted to the ventricles.

A narrow QRS complex suggests that the block is high in the AV junction. A broad QRS complex suggests a lower block, which may have more serious connotations and may forewarn of more dangerous arrhythmias.

With a very slow ventricular rate, the patient may have symptoms such as dizziness, blackouts, angina or breathlessness. Atropine or isoprenaline are sometimes used to try to improve the ventricular rate and temporary pacing may be required, particularly with the broad complex form of the arrhythmia.

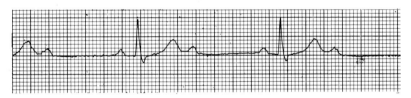

Fig. 7.4 Second degree AV block — Mobitz type II, 2:1. Note that the PR interval is constant and just within the normal limits of duration (0.20 seconds).

Differentiation between the Second Degree AV Blocks

It is often very difficult to differentiate between Wenckebach phenomenon and Mobitz type II second degree AV block. Indeed in type II (2:1 block), it is not possible to say whether the PR interval would have lengthened, had there been more conducted beats. In any case, the PR intervals should be examined carefully on a rhythm strip before a diagnosis is made.

Third Degree AV Block

Third degree AV block is also called complete heart block. It is

generally more serious than first and second degree blocks. It is characterised by complete absence of conduction between the atria and ventricles so they beat independently from each other. On the ECG monitor there appears a series of P waves at a normal, regular rate as SA node impulse formation and conduction are not impaired. However, none of these impulses are conducted to the ventricles. Ventricular pacemakers tend to produce slower, regular ventricular depolarisation. If the ventricular pacemaker is high (for example, in the bundle of His), the QRS complexes produced will be narrow and of a reasonable rate; if the ventricular pacemaker is low (for example, in the Purkinje fibres), the QRS complexes will be broad and the inherent rate very slow.

On the ECG monitor, the ventricular rhythm bears no relationship to that of the atria although both are regular. There are many more P waves than QRS complexes. The PR interval is constantly changing (Fig. 7.5).

If the ventricular rate is very slow, the patient will often suffer from dizzy spells or even blackouts (Stokes–Adams attacks). Angina and breathlessness may also be encountered. Complete heart block may lead to ventricular irritability and dangerous rapid ventricular arrhythmias; sometimes it may precede ventricular standstill if the ventricular pacemaker is unreliable. It is common for patients suffering from complete heart block to require temporary pacemaker insertion to relieve their symptoms and prevent more dangerous events occurring. The need for permanent pacing can then be assessed. Isoprenaline therapy is sometimes commenced intravenously to increase ventricular heart rate and contractility until temporary pacing can be performed. Slow release isoprenaline may be given orally on a long-term basis if pacing is inappropriate.

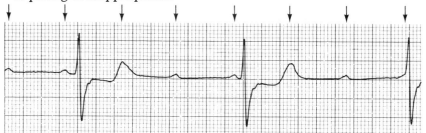

Fig. 7.5 Complete heart block. The atrial rate is approximately 100. The ventricular rate is 33. Some of the P waves are hidden in the T waves. Arrows indicate position of P waves.

Ventricular Standstill

Ventricular standstill may occur following junctional or intraventricular conduction defects where the ventricular pacemaker is
unreliable. Effective electrical stimulation and conduction continue in the atria but cease in the ventricles. On the ECG, P waves
continue normally but there are no QRS complexes (Fig. 7.6).
Ventricular standstill is a life-threatening situation and cardiopulmonary resuscitation must be performed until facilities for pacing
are made available. This is referred to as primary ventricular
standstill by some authorities (Meltzer, Pinneo and Kitchell,
1977).

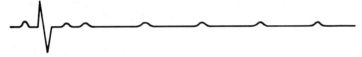

Fig. 7.6   Ventricular standstill.

AV Dissociation

The term AV dissociation may be used to describe any rhythm
where the atria and ventricles are operating independently of each
other. However, the term is also often applied to the situation
which mimics AV block, caused by competition between atrial
and ventricular pacemakers, rather than an organic lesion. The
atria are depolarised by an atrial pacemaker which may be the SA
node. The ventricles are depolarised by a junctional or high
ventricular pacemaker, which discharges at a rate similar to that of
the atrial pacemaker.

The atrial impulse cannot be conducted through the AV junction to the ventricles as these areas have already been stimulated
and made refractory by the ventricular pacemaker. Neither can
the ventricular pacemaker cause retrograde stimulation, as the
atria have been stimulated by their own pacemaker. As the timing
of the pacemakers is constantly changing slightly, the situation
eventually arises when the atrial impulse can be conducted
through the AV junction to capture the ventricles. This beat is
called a 'capture' beat and may temporarily revert the AV dissociation to sinus rhythm.

AV dissociation rarely requires treatment as the ventricular rate is usually good. However, the cause for the speeding up of the ventricular pacemaker or slowing of the SA node should be sought. Digoxin therapy and acute myocardial infarction are well known as causes of these effects.

On the ECG, the P waves and the QRS complexes of AV dissociation bear no relationship to each other, although the rates of both are similar. The P waves are often described as 'marching through' the QRS complexes. The PR interval becomes progressively shorter and the P wave eventually disappears within the QRS complex before emerging on the other side. Capture beats appear as normal sinus beats.

CONDUCTION DEFECTS ARISING IN THE RIGHT AND LEFT BUNDLE BRANCHES

Initial ventricular depolarisation normally starts in the left side of the interventricular septum, activating it from left to right. The ECG will therefore show an upward deflection, or small r wave, in

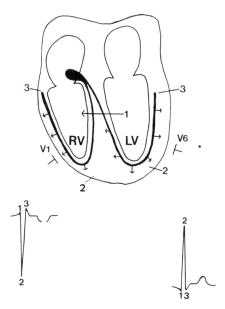

Fig. 7.7 Normal ventricular depolarisation: 1. from left to right across the septum; 2. depolarisation of main ventricular walls (endocardium to epicardium); 3. base of ventricular walls.

the right chest leads. A small downward deflection, or q wave, is seen over the left chest leads (Fig. 7.7). Depolarisation of the ventricles then occurs simultaneously but the left ventricle is more dominant because of its larger size. The resultant ventricular vector is therefore from right to left. The right chest leads will show a deep S wave following the small initial r wave; the left chest leads will record a tall R wave following the q wave deflection (Fig. 7.7).

Right Bundle Branch Block (RBBB)

In RBBB, conduction through the right bundle branch of the bundle of His is impeded. Depolarisation proceeds normally down the left bundle branch and crosses the interventricular septum from left to right. Thus the initial vector of the QRS complex is normal. Thereafter the impulse proceeds swiftly and normally to the left ventricle resulting in an S wave in V_1 and V_2 and an R wave in V_5 and V_6. However, depolarisation of the right ventricle is delayed as the right bundle branch is blocked. It is eventually depolarised later when the impulse from the left ventricle reaches it, via the ordinary myocardium. This results in an R wave in V_1 and V_2 and an S wave in V_5 and V_6. The delay results in a broad QRS complex (over 0·10 seconds) which is notched, indicating individual rather than simultaneous ventricular depolarisation (Fig. 7.8). Figure 7.9 shows the ECG of a patient with RBBB.

Fig. 7.8   QRS configuration in the right and left chest leads in RBBB.

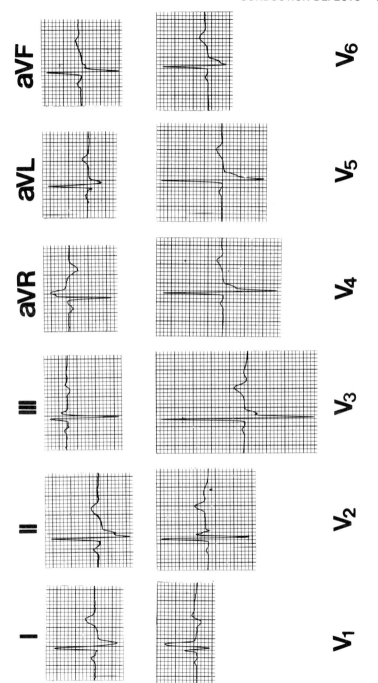

Fig. 7.9   The ECG of a patient with RBBB.

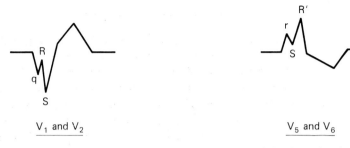

Fig. 7.10   QRS configuration in the right and left chest leads in LBBB.

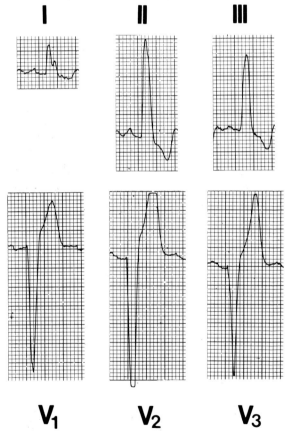

Fig. 7.11   The ECG of a patient with LBBB.

Left Bundle Branch Block (LBBB)

In LBBB conduction through the left bundle branch is impeded. Depolarisation cannot proceed normally through the interventricular septum. Septal depolarisation occurs from the healthy right bundle, resulting in alteration of the initial vector of the QRS complex. Next, the right ventricle depolarises, but left ventricular depolarisation is delayed until the impulse spreads to it from the right ventricle. This results in a qRS complex in V_1 and V_2 and an rSR pattern in V_5 and V_6. Again, the complexes produced are broad and often notched, indicating the separate depolarisation of the two ventricles (Fig. 7.10). The LBBB pattern often masks the ECG changes of myocardial infarction. Figure 7.11 shows the

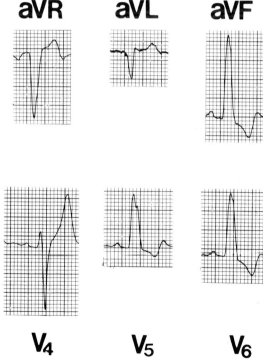

Fig. 7.11   Contd.

ECG of a patient with LBBB. RBBB may occur as a normal variant in certain individuals. Other causes are pulmonary emboli, ischaemic heart disease, right ventricular overload, cardiomyopathy, rheumatic heart disease, viral infections of the heart and atrial septal defects.

LBBB is commonly associated with ischaemic heart disease, hypertension, aortic stenosis, hypertropic obstructive cardiomyopathy, rheumatic fever, myocarditis, syphilis, cardiac tumours, cardiac surgery and congenital heart disease. The treatment depends on the cause of the block. LBBB is generally more serious than RBBB.

Hemiblock and Bifascicular Block

The left bundle branch divides into two main fascicles, one passing anteriorly and the other posteriorly.

When a block occurs in one of these fascicles (hemiblock), the change may be diagnosed by the shift of electrical axis. Block in the anterior fascicle (left anterior hemiblock) results in left axis deviation, whereas block in the posterior fascicle (left posterior hemiblock) results in right axis deviation. If a RBBB occurs with a left anterior hemiblock or left posterior hemiblock, then bifascicular block is said to occur. The situation may result from anterior myocardial infarction.

When two fascicles supplying the ventricles are blocked, there is only one remaining operational conduction pathway. Should infarction extend or ischaemia worsen, the third fascicle may also block, resulting in complete heart block or ventricular standstill.

Temporary pacing may be required when bifascicular block occurs following acute myocardial infarction. Permanent pacing will be required if it is the result of chronic fibrosis of the conducting system.

Further Reading

Andreoli K.G., Hunn–Fowkes V., Zipes D.P., Wallace A.G. (1979). Arrhythmias. In *Comprehensive Cardiac Care: a Text for Nurses, Physicians and Other Health Practitioners*, 4th edn., pp.128–257. St. Louis: The C.V. Mosby Company.

de Bono D. (1982). Funny Turns. *British Journal of Hospital Medicine;* 27:212–223.

Meltzer L.E., Pinneo R., Kitchell J.R. (1977). Disorders of Conduction and Ventricular Standstill. In *Intensive Coronary Care: a manual for nurses*. 3rd edn., pp.193–208 and pp.209–213. Bowie, Md.: The Charles Press Publishers.

Rowlands D.J. (1982). Morphological abnormalities. In *Understanding the Electrocardiogram*. pp.110–143. Macclesfield: Imperial Chemical Industries PLC.

Schamroth L. (1976). *An Introduction to Electrocardiography*, 5th edn. Oxford: Blackwell Scientific Publications.

Wade E.G. (1982). Symptomless abnormalities, minor ECG abnormalities. *British Journal of Hospital Medicine;* **27**:615–623.

8

Pacemakers

A pacemaker system consists of a wire or electrode which is inserted into the heart and attached to a battery operated pacing box. This is set to deliver timed electrical impulses to the heart. In a temporary pacing system, the box is situated externally (Fig. 8.1); in a permanent system, it is implanted within the subcutaneous tissue of the body (Fig. 8.2). On the ECG, paced beats resemble ventricular ectopics preceded by a spike which represents the pacing stimulus (Fig. 8.3).

Temporary Pacemakers — Reasons for Insertion

There are many indications for pacemaker insertion. Temporary pacemakers are usually inserted for therapeutic reasons but are also widely used as an aid to diagnosis. The most common reasons for temporary pacemaker insertion are:

1. to provide reliable electrical stimulation to the heart in the presence of conduction abnormalities associated with myocardial infarction.
2. to treat any situation where transient reduced heart rate is causing life-threatening symptoms, e.g. blackouts.
3. as a prophylactic measure after cardiac surgery.
4. when a cardiac arrest is caused by extreme bradycardia or asystole and is not responding to drug treatment.
5. to treat certain tachyarrhythmias by overdrive or underdrive pacing.

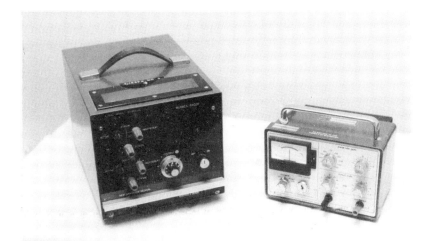

Fig. 8.1 Two examples of temporary pacing boxes. On the left is the Sussex box, one of the prototypes of the synchronous pacing boxes. On the right is a demand pacing box with the special 'times 3' mode for underdrive/overdrive pacing. (The picture of the Sussex box is published by kind permission of Dr D. Chamberlain, The Royal Sussex Hospital, Brighton).

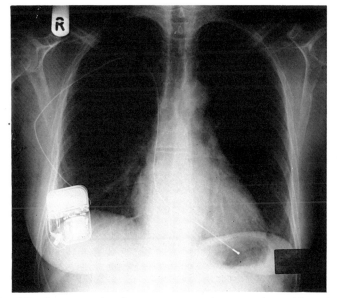

Fig. 8.2 An x-ray showing a permanent pacemaker with a right ventricular endocardial pacing wire.

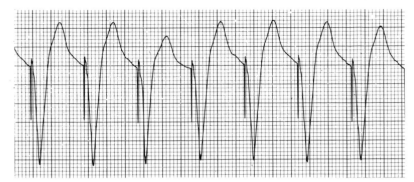

Fig. 8.3 Continuous ventricular pacing showing prominent pacing spikes.

6. as an aid to diagnosis.

The most frequently used temporary pacing electrode has two poles situated on the catheter itself (bipolar). The unipolar electrode has one pole on the electrode, the other neutral or indifferent pole being attached to the pacing box. The unipolar electrode is usually used in permanent pacing systems. Other commercially produced catheters may have three, four or six poles. These are used for electrophysiology studies.

Permanent Pacemakers — Reasons for Insertion

Permanent pacemakers are always inserted for therapeutic reasons, the most common of which are listed below:

1. when a conduction abnormality which was thought to be transient does not return to normal during adequate assessment with a temporary system.
2. for complete heart block which is permanent or intermittent and from which the patient is getting symptoms such as Stokes–Adams attacks.
3. for sick-sinus syndrome, characterised by episodes of tachycardia and bradycardia.
4. in some centres, permanent pacing is performed when bifascicular block persists after myocardial infarction. For these patients the prognosis is poor, but may be slightly improved by permanent pacing.

5. specially programmable permanent pacemakers are now available for the termination of paroxysmal tachycardias.

METHODS OF INSERTION

Transvenous and transthoracic routes are commonly employed for pacemaker insertion.

Temporary Pacing — Transvenous Approach

A peripheral vein such as the femoral, jugular, subclavian or antecubital is usually used for transvenous insertion of a temporary pacing electrode. A percutaneous approach or cut-down procedure can be employed. The pacing wire is threaded from the peripheral vein into the right atrium, through the tricuspid valve and on into the right ventricle. With the help of x-ray screening, its tip is positioned on the endocardium at the ventricular apex. The patient is asked to cough and take some deep breaths to make sure the wire is stable before the electrical threshold is checked. The threshold is defined as the minimum amount of electricity required to depolarise the heart reliably. If the position of the electrode tip is good, the threshold should be less than 1 mv. The pacing box can then be set at the desired heart rate, with the voltage setting at least twice the threshold level to allow for possible threshold alterations. The pacing wire is sutured to the skin at the site of entry and a sterile dressing applied. An x-ray is usually taken to check the position of the electrode and to exclude pneumothorax if the subclavian route has been used. The transvenous approach can also be used for atrial pacing when a temporary pacing wire is situated in the right atrium. This may be used for patients with normal AV conduction and sinus bradycardia. Atrial pacing (Fig. 8.4) preserves the synchrony of the atria

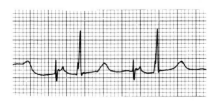

Fig. 8.4   Atrial pacing.

and ventricles, resulting in better cardiac output than that achieved by ventricular pacing.

Temporary Pacing — Transthoracic Approach

A transthoracic approach may be used for temporary pacing procedures. When emergency pacing is required during a cardiac arrest, a wire is inserted through the left chest wall into the cavity of the left ventricle. Gentle traction ensures contact with the endocardium. An external pacing box can then be used to pass electrical stimuli along the wire and stimulate the ventricle. This procedure is potentially hazardous, but may be life-saving. The electrode is unstable, especially if external cardiac massage is used. If it produces beneficial effects, it must be replaced by a temporary transvenous electrode as soon as possible.

Temporary transthoracic pacemakers are also commonly implanted following cardiac surgery. The wire is attached to the epicardium and brought out through the incision in the chest wall. Transthoracic wires can be used if arrhythmias arise or if postoperative electrophysiology studies are anticipated.

Permanent Pacing — Transvenous Approach

When a permanent pacing procedure is performed, an electrode may be passed transvenously through the subclavian or jugular vein and onwards through the right side of the heart to rest in the apex of the right ventricle. The other end of the wire is tunnelled through the subcutaneous tissues and attached to the small permanent box which is implanted in the chest wall.

Permanent Pacing — Transthoracic Approach

The transthoracic approach may also be employed for permanent pacemakers. This may be necessary if repeated attempts with a transvenous approach have failed to give a stable right ventricular position or if a thoracic operation is being performed for some other reason and a permanent pacemaker is also required. Until recently it has been the preferred route for pacing children, because of problems with growth. After thoracotomy, the distal end of the electrode is sutured or clipped onto the epicardium, the other end being directed through the subcutaneous tissues to the site chosen for implantation of the permanent box. This is usually the abdominal wall or supramammary region.

Pacemaker Batteries

Many types of battery cells have been used for permanent pacemaker systems over the years, such as mercury, zinc and nickel. Lithium batteries have gained popularity and are now widely used. They do not corrode and have a rate of battery depletion which can be predicted fairly reliably, some units lasting for 12 years or more.

The rate and voltage of temporary pacemakers can be adjusted on the external box as desired. The rate and voltage of permanent pacemakers are usually preset by the manufacturers although programmable pacemakers have been introduced recently, allowing these parameters to be altered externally.

MODES OF ACTION OF PACEMAKERS

Pacemakers may operate:

1. at a fixed rate or
2. on demand.

Fixed Rate Pacemakers

Pacemakers set on the fixed rate mode will deliver continuous regular electrical stimuli at the set voltage, regardless of any naturally occurring stimuli produced by the heart. Competition sometimes occurs between the natural and artificial stimuli and may produce ventricular arrhythmias. It is for this reason that the fixed rate pacing mode has lost popularity.

Demand Pacemakers

Pacemakers set on the demand mode deliver stimuli to the heart only when the natural pacemakers produce or conduct impulses at a slower rate than that set on the pacing box. Thus, when the ventricular rate slows, the artificial pacemakers will deliver stimuli at the predetermined rate, rather like an escape rhythm.

If the patient's own heart rate recovers, the pacemaker senses it and further pacing impulses are inhibited.

Ventricular demand pacing is the most common type of pacing used today. Competition between the natural and artificial pacemakers should not occur although fusion beats may arise due to late firing of the natural pacemaker coinciding with the artificial stimuli.

Other Modes of Pacing

In the above forms of pacing there is no synchrony between the atria and ventricles. In certain situations it is desirable to maintain synchrony to improve cardiac output. Pacing which preserves AV synchrony is commonly referred to as 'physiological pacing'. It can be achieved by either:

1. triggering the ventricular pacemaker from the P waves (synchronous pacing), or
2. pacing both the atria and the ventricles in sequence (sequential pacing).

Both these modes of pacing require atrial and ventricular electrodes (Fig. 8.5).

Synchronous Pacing

In P wave-triggered synchronous pacing, the atrial electrode allows atrial depolarisation to be sensed. A preset time interval occurs before ventricular depolarisation is produced by the ventricular pacing electrode. Thus a normal PR interval is mimicked. If no P wave is present the ventricular pacemaker will nevertheless produce artificial ventricular stimuli at a set rate. A blocking device prevents the pacemaker from following rapid supraventricular arrhythmias.

AV Sequential Pacing

In AV sequential pacing, the atrial electrode not only senses but can also pace the atrium. Ventricular pacing is then triggered by the atrial pacing stimulus. This would be valuable in situations where sinus node and AV node conduction abnormalities coexist (Fig. 8.6).

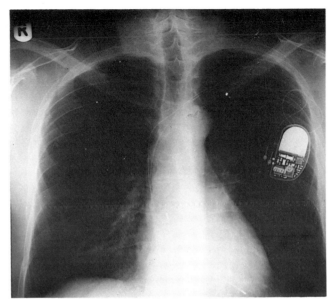

Fig. 8.5   An implanted AV sequential pacemaker showing atrial and ventricular wires.

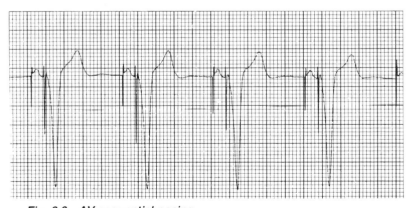

Fig. 8.6   AV sequential pacing.

NURSING CARE OF PATIENTS WITH PACEMAKERS

Temporary Pacemakers — Nursing Care

The nurse has an important role to play before, during and after insertion of a temporary pacing electrode. A check list for the preparation of the patient before the procedure is given below:

1. Explain the procedure to the patient and relatives.
2. Ensure consent is signed.
3. Fast the patient for a few hours if possible.
4. Shave the site to be used for electrode insertion.
5. Note any allergies, e.g. to the iodine-based skin cleaning solution, drugs, elastoplast.
6. Check patient identity.
7. Dress as for theatre in gown; remove jewellery and dentures.
8. Record temperature, heart and respiratory rate, and blood pressure. Monitor heart rhythm continuously.
9. Allow patient to pass urine just before the procedure.

The room and equipment for the procedure must be organised and the resuscitation trolley placed near at hand. X-ray technicians often have to be alerted to screen the procedure.

During electrode insertion, the nurse must assist the doctor while at the same time observing the monitor and ensuring the comfort of the patient. When a good electrode position is achieved, the wire is attached to the pacing box by red and black extension leads and the threshold checked. The box is then set at the desired heart rate and voltage, the wire is sutured into position and a dressing is applied. All connections are rechecked; the patient is transferred back to his own room and made comfortable in bed before the equipment is cleared away.

Following the procedure, the nurse's responsibilities fall into three main categories:

1. the physical comfort of the patient.
2. the technical care of the equipment.
3. the psychological well-being of the patient and his relatives.

Physical care

The patient may feel much better physically following the pacing procedure. However, analgesia or sedation may be required. Mobility will be restricted; the length of time in bed will depend on the cause of the conduction disturbance. General hygiene must be taken care of meticulously during this time, with a daily bed bath and regular care to pressure areas, mouth and hair. Often the patient may eat and drink what he wants, although on occasions there may be restrictions.

The pacemaker insertion site must be regularly observed for signs of infection, bleeding and thrombophlebitis. The sterile dressing should be changed as often as required for the patient's comfort. The patency and sites of any other intravenous or arterial lines must also be observed frequently.

If a urinary catheter is inserted, catheter toilet is necessary. Use of the commode is permitted, but care must be taken not to dislodge the pacing electrode. Aperients may be required to prevent constipation. Regular passive exercises in bed are encouraged to prevent complications of bed rest.

Observations of blood pressure, heart rate and rhythm are extremely important after pacing electrode insertion and may be required every half hour initially. Temperature and respiratory rate should also be recorded regularly. Medication is given as prescribed by the medical staff.

The Technical Care of the Equipment

There are certain technical aspects of patient care which are important after a pacing procedure. Continuous cardiac monitoring is required for observation of arrhythmias. A 12 lead electrocardiograph should be recorded as soon as possible. The box settings of heart rate, voltage and mode of pacing are documented in the nursing kardex. Checks on the connections between the patient, electrode and box are made routinely to ensure that they have not become loose or detached. Daily checks of the batteries should also be made when temporary pacing boxes are being used. The threshold levels must be measured and documented twice daily; at these times, the patient's underlying rhythm can also be assessed. This is usually performed by experienced nursing staff, but the medical staff may prefer to make these checks if the patient is prone to life-threatening arrhythmias. If possible, routine daily ECGs should be performed with the pacing box switched off. Other points of note to the nurse are:

1. the extension leads should be secured to the limb, to prevent excess pulling and possible displacement of the electrode itself. The splinting of a limb may also be necessary.

2.   the ends of multi-pole electrodes (e.g. hexipolar wires) which
     are not in use should be bound lightly with tape to prevent
     short circuiting or transmission of static electricity.
3.   the temporary box should be attached securely to the patient's
     clothes or a limb, or to the bed if the patient is confined to it. It
     should never be left on the floor or bedside locker where it
     may get kicked or knocked over.
4.   if defibrillation is required, the pacing box should be switched
     off while it is performed.

Psychological Care

The psychological care of the patient and relatives is very important. Simple unhurried explanations about the pacemaker will
reassure them, restore their confidence and help to gain their
cooperation.

Removal

If the patient regains normal heart rhythm, the medical staff will
request that the temporary pacing electrode is removed. This
aseptic procedure can be carried out at the patient's bedside by a
nurse or doctor. The procedure is explained to the patient and the
box is switched off and detached from the leads and electrode. The
suture is cut and the wire is withdrawn gently. The monitor is
observed for evidence of any irritability of the heart caused by the
procedure. A sterile dressing is applied to the site. The patient
may feel apprehensive without the pacemaker and may require a
good deal of reassurance and encouragement at this time.

Some pacing electrodes can be resterilised, but many are dispos-
able and should not be reused.

Permanent Pacemakers — Nursing Care

The preparation of a patient for permanent pacemaker insertion is
not unlike that for a temporary pacemaker. However, there are
several additional points to be remembered:

1.   more time is often available prior to insertion, so it should be
     possible to fast the patient for 6 hours if the procedure is to be
     done under local anaesthetic and for 12 hours if the patient is
     to have a general anaesthetic for thoracotomy.
2.   a greater area of the body should be shaved — arms, axilla and

chest for an endocardial system, neck to knees for an epicardial device.
3. height and weight should be measured and recorded.
4. patient identity should be checked in detail.
5. a premedication may be prescribed.
6. the patient is usually transferred to theatre for the procedure and should be accompanied by a nurse, who takes with her the patient's x-rays, hospital notes and drug chart.

After permanent pacing the patient is transferred back to the ward and made comfortable in bed. Analgesia may be required. A chest x-ray and an electrocardiograph are performed. Bed rest is required for approximately 24 hours during which time continuous cardiac monitoring is carried out to observe the action of the pacemaker. The patient should be advised not to lift his arms above his shoulders during the first day, as this may dislodge the box. Assistance with general hygiene is necessary. The site of the permanent box should be observed daily for haematoma, bleeding, cellulitis or infection, and dressings should be renewed as often as required.

A redivac drain may be inserted during the operation; it can usually be removed the next day if bleeding is not excessive. Observations of temperature, pulse, respiratory rate and blood pressure are carried out every 4 hours unless there is an indication for more frequent recordings.

Food and fluids can be taken freely after a local anaesthetic, although restrictions will follow a general anaesthetic.

The mode of pacing and box type number should be recorded after permanent pacemaker insertion.

Many incisions are repaired with absorbable subcuticular stitches. If non-absorbable sutures are present, they should be removed about seven days after the operation. However, discharge from hospital need not be delayed as this can be done by the district nurse.

Psychological Care

Good psychological care of the patient and his relatives can go a long way to re-establish an independent and enjoyable life-style. Reassurance is necessary that an active life is possible. Permanent pacemakers are reliable. They have known battery run-down dates, so patients can be admitted for replacements before symptoms are encountered. In addition, patients will have regular electrocardiographs and reassessments of the pacemaker system. Telephone systems are in use in some centres to allow for easy pacemaker assessments without the patient having to travel long distances to a cardiology centre. With this device, the patient's electrocardiograph can be transmitted to the relevant department where it is analysed by the medical staff.

Other advice is needed by patients — how to take their pulse and what to do if it is outside certain limits. Significant slowing may suggest impending battery run-down. The dangers of micro-wave ovens, fairground dodgem cars and airport safety devices should be emphasised, as should the need to reapply for a new driving licence.

Every patient with a permanent pacemaker is given a card with the pacemaker details on it. He should be advised to carry this with him at all times. He should also be advised to tell his doctor or dentist about his pacemaker before he accepts any treatment.

COMPLICATIONS OF PACEMAKERS

Complications are relatively rare. However, problems do arise occasionally, and nursing and medical staff must be alert for them.

There are several complications which relate to pacemaker insertion. Pneumothorax and pulmonary emboli are possible, and infection may take the form of abscess formation, septicaemia or, more rarely, endocarditis. Bleeding may occur at the site. Right ventricular perforation may result in pericardial friction rub or diaphragmatic stimulation by the pacing wire and may be associated with cardiac tamponade. Occasionally, the wire perforates the ventricular septum causing a change in the conduction pattern from a left bundle branch block pattern to that of a right. With permanent systems, the electrodes or boxes may erode overlying tissues, in which case they will need to be repositioned.

Other complications relate to problems of pacing or sensing. With permanent systems, battery failure is probably the most common complication and may result in reduced pacing rate, failure to discharge an impulse or failure to produce a stimulus of sufficient voltage to cause ventricular depolarisation. Fractured electrodes or loose connections may cause pacing failure. Abnormal firing may also occur when parts of the pacemaker's system fail. This 'runaway' pacemaker is serious and may lead to ventricular fibrillation. The electrode must be disconnected from the pacing box immediately if this situation arises. Fibrosis at the tip of a catheter which has been in position for some time may prevent the pacing stimulus from depolarising the heart. This often requires the insertion of a new electrode.

When a pacing box fails to sense the patient's own electrical impulses, it will discharge irrespective of these and set up a competitive rhythm. Wire displacement may be the reason for this, or the electrode may be lying on an area of tissue which is ischaemic or infarcted and thus electrically inert. Oversensing may occur when a pacemaker senses signals other than ventricular depolarisation and thus suppresses required pacing impulses. Generally, epicardial wires are more stable and less prone to displacement than those inserted transvenously.

Nursing and medical staff must be familiar with the mechanics of pacing electrodes, boxes and paced rhythms. Abnormalities or problems observed by the nursing staff must be reported immediately.

Further Reading

Andreoli K.G., Hunn–Fowkes V., Zipes D.P., Wallace A.G. (1979). Artificial Cardiac Pacemakers. In *Comprehensive Cardiac Care: a Text for Nurses, Physicians and Other Health Practitioners*, 4th edn., pp.258–279. St. Louis: The C.V. Mosby Company.

de Bono D. (1982). Funny Turns. *British Journal of Hospital Medicine;* 27:212–223.

Donaldson R.M., Fox K., Rickards A.F. (1983). Initial experience with a physiological, rate responsive pacemaker. *British Medical Journal;* 286:667–671.

Hayward R. (1981). Who do we pace? *British Journal of Hospital Medicine;* 25:466–474.

Meltzer L.E., Pinneo R., Kitchell J.R. (1977). The Electrical Treatment of Arrhythmias. In *Intensive Coronary Care: a manual for nurses*, 3rd edn., pp.215–229. Bowie, Md.: The Charles Press Publishers.

O'Brien G.J. (1979). The nursing care of patients with cardiac pacemakers. *Nursing Times;* 75(4): 147–151.

Radford D.J., Julian D.G. (1974). Sick Sinus Syndrome: Experience of a Cardiac Pacemaker Clinic. *British Medical Journal;* 3:504–507.

Thompson D,R. (1982). Ischaemic heart disease. In *Cardiac Nursing*, 1st edn., pp.133–205. London: Baillière Tindall.

Waller S. (1982). Pacemakers. *Nursing Times;* 78:941–943.

9

Psychological Aspects

The majority of patients admitted to the CCU undergo varying degrees of emotional stress. This is a normal response to myocardial infarction and subsequent hospitalisation. It is important that the team caring for these patients can recognise and treat these responses early in the CCU as psychological problems can impair progress and rehabilitation.

In the early hours following myocardial infarction, anxiety and fear of death are the natural responses — the severe chest pain, the immediate transfer to hospital and the admission to the strange and perhaps frightening environment of CCU may add to the stress. Increase in sympathetic drive may result in further pain, arrhythmias and subsequent cardiac failure. The prompt management of pain is essential; usually morphine 10 mg or diamorphine 5 mg is given intravenously with an anti-emetic such as prochlorperazine 12·5 mg or metoclorpromide 10 mg. Together with reassurance from calm and confident staff, this will do much to alleviate fear. It is the CCU staff who will begin the psychological management and rehabilitation of the patient and this care should also extend to include the relatives.

Once the patient is over the initial crisis, his anxiety may revolve around his future and may be due to apprehension regarding his occupation and socio-economic status. This anxiety may affect his relationships with his family and with society at large. In particular, it may occur when a change in occupation is necessary or advisable as will be the case with airline pilots, miners and long-distance lorry drivers of heavy goods vehicles. In these cases the rehabilitation officer should visit; the social worker can also be of great help. This help should be sought sooner rather than later. Occasionally anxiety and fear in a patient is not easily appreciated and may only be realised if the patient develops a sinus tachycardia or is restless and unable to relax. He may develop an unusual exaggerated curiosity in his illness. It may be necessary to prescribe an anxiolytic drug such as diazepam orally.

Sometimes patients respond to the illness by denial — they do not accept they have had a heart attack. These patients show a mood of unusual optimism and tend to deny any symptoms. They try to mobilise too early, particularly during the early phase of rehabilitation, to prove to themselves that they are the same person as before they were admitted to hospital.

A patient may react in anger to his infarct — he asks himself why it should have happened to him and looks around for the answer. He may blame stress at work, family situations or the family doctor and this may show in his attitude towards the staff.

Some patients react by becoming depressed on being admitted to the CCU — they see their life as over and become tearful and withdrawn. The patient becomes totally dependent on those who care for him and may even expect his wife to wait on him. Reassurance and encouragement is of particular importance to depressed patients and their relatives.

The patient's transfer from the CCU to the main ward may be a source of worry to him as he may feel vulnerable because he is less closely supervised. Encouragement from the staff with emphasis on rehabilitation and on discharge to home will do much to alleviate concern. In some hospitals the CCU staff follow their patients' progress in the main ward, giving continuity to their care. Women suffer the same psychological problems as men, but have additional worries. For example, wives often fear initially that their families will be unable to cope without them. Later, paradoxically, a woman may feel useless and unneeded when she hears that her household is managing perfectly well. This situation obviously requires tactful handling by the staff and the husband.

Relatives

Relatives undergo a great deal of stress at this time. Communication with both medical and nursing staff is constantly encouraged;

anxious relatives can add further stress to an already stressful situation. If the medical and nursing staff can anticipate responses to stress and if they emphasise that these are normal reactions to illness, it will help both patients and relatives to come to terms with illness and to look forward to the future. It should be appreciated by both medical and nursing staff that relatives need to be seen frequently and to have frequent explanations of progress. Often the same explanation may have to be repeated several times as relatives fail to understand what they have been told initially in the stress of the situation. Finally it should be realised by both patient and by relatives that even after discharge, the patient may be susceptible to mood swings during the early days, which if not understood can add to tension in family life.

Some patients and relatives derive benefit from joining a local organisation which provides social interaction and practical projects with people who have had similar experiences, e.g. the British Heart Foundation.

Further Reading

Andreoli K.G., Hunn–Fowkes V., Zipes D.P., Wallace A.G. (1979). Care of the Cardiac Patient. In *Comprehensive Cardiac Care; a Text for Nurses, Physicians and Other Health Practitioners*, 4th edn., pp.311–317. St. Louis: The C.V. Mosby Company.

Denolin H. (1982). *Psychological problems — before and after myocardial infarction*. Basel: S. Karger.

Gentry W.D., Williams R.B. (1979). *Psychological aspects of myocardial infarction and coronary care*. 2nd edn. St. Louis. The C.V. Mosby Company Ltd.

Meltzer L.E., Pinneo R., Kitchell J. (1977). *Intensive Coronary Care: a Manual for Nurses*, 3rd edn., pp.70–73. Bowie, Md.: The Charles Press Publishers.

Sime A.M. (1983). Lessening patient stress in the CCU. *Nursing Management;* **14** (1):24–26.

Solomon–Hast A. (1981). Anxiety in the coronary care unit: assessment and intervention. *Critical Care Quarterly;* **4**:75–82.

10

Rehabilitation and Secondary Prevention

REHABILITATION

According to the Oxford English Dictionary, the term 'rehabilitation' was introduced during the reign of Henry VIII and used in the context of the rehabilitation and restoration of possessions and lands to their original owners. The word 'rehabilitation' as we know it, however, was first used just before the Second World War and described to the conditioning and welfare of miners suffering from industrial injury. It was subsequently associated with trauma and other medical disorders.

'Cardiac' rehabilitation is a total programme designed to promote desirable changes in life pattern through education, counselling and exercise which will return the patient to his place in society. Counselling also includes the family. The majority of patients following myocardial infarction will return to work in six to eight weeks.

In 1964 coronary rehabilitation of patients was described by the World Health Organisation as 'the sum of activity required to ensure the best possible physical, mental and social conditions so that they may, by their own efforts, regain as normal as possible a place in the community and lead an active productive life' (WHO, 1964). In 1975 a joint Royal College of Physicians working party under the chairmanship of Thomas Semple, produced a report on rehabilitation of the coronary patient. The working party examined the problems associated with coronary artery disease and considered the physical, psychological, social and economic aspects of rehabilitation. The report hoped to stimulate good practice with further research into the subject. Since that report and others which followed, much has been achieved to return the patient to work and reintegrate him into society as quickly as possible. It is commonly acknowledged that patients with coronary artery disease are invalided for unnecessarily prolonged periods and that this may be the result of depression, anxiety, social difficulties or even inadequate medical management.

Rehabilitation begins in the CCU. It is here that relationships with medical and nursing staff are established. During the acute stage of myocardial infarction, the emphasis is on the management of pain, cardiac failure and arrhythmias. However it is also during this stage that explanations to the patient and his relatives, about the immediate events and surroundings as well as what to expect in the future, are very important. The role of the staff in the CCU is to help the patient to come to terms with his illness, prepare him for his transfer to the ward and for his future life, in addition to giving support to the family.

The many aspects of rehabilitation in the progressive coronary care unit are discussed in Chapters 5 and 9.

SECONDARY PREVENTION

Secondary prevention can be regarded as the next logical step following rehabilitation. Its aim is to prevent the progression of coronary artery disease, relieve symptoms and improve prognosis.

Education

Education is the cornerstone of secondary prevention. It should begin as soon as coronary artery disease is diagnosed.

Smoking

Advice is necessary for the patient and his family about the risks of continuing to smoke; studies have shown that patients who have stopped smoking have a lower mortality rate than those who continue with the habit. Some patients find it difficult to stop smoking but helpful booklets are available from the Health

Education Council, the address of which is given below:

> The Health Education Council
> 78, New Oxford Street
> London
> WC1A 1AH

Special information packs have now been designed by the Health Education Council to help nurses educate their patients about smoking. Television programmes and the mass media campaign against smoking but perhaps the best way that nurses can assist patients to stop the habit is to enlist the help of and to motivate the whole family.

Diet

Most patients being admitted to the CCU will not require special diets but will be advised to eat good healthy food. Much emphasis is now placed on eating wholesome foods not only for those who are at risk of heart disease but for the general population as a whole. Healthy food should promote good health and is a primary means of preventing disease.

The overweight are advised to keep to a calorie controlled diet which may require the supervision of a dietician. The value of reducing lipid levels is a controversial subject except in young patients with familial hyperlipidaemia. Patients may also need to reduce their alcohol intake if this is excessive. However, moderate consumption of alcohol is acceptable for those who are not overweight.

Exercise

Exercise programmes are encouraged for patients with coronary artery disease and many hospitals organise formal exercise sessions. Here patients participate in supervised and graded exercise and have social contact with people who have similar problems. However, too often exercise is thought to be the basis of rehabilitation and secondary prevention. This is not so; exercise is just part of the total programme. Even without organised exercise programmes, patients can discipline themselves to take regular daily exercise thus altering their previous sedentary life-style.

Exercise Tests

Modified exercise tests are organised for many patients before discharge from hospital. A further exercise test is arranged six weeks later and as well as being a psychological boost for patients who do well, it is a useful prognostic aid for the cardiologist regarding management which may include coronary artery bypass grafts.

Stress

Patients require much psychological support after myocardial infarction (Chapter 9). They need help to come to terms with their illness and the limitations it imposes on their life style. Fatigue and mood swings are common. If possible some of the stresses of a hectic life pattern should be removed.

Medical Management

It is important that patients understand the necessity for medical follow-up after myocardial infarction. Out-patient appointments are usually arranged for approximately one month after discharge. Thereafter, care may be continued at the hospital on an out-patient basis or it may be taken over by the family doctor. By regular check-ups, risk factors which may predispose people to further myocardial infarction can be carefully monitored. Hypertension is a major risk factor of coronary artery disease and must be carefully controlled. Patients with diabetes must also be closely observed as this condition makes them prone to disease of the coronary arteries.

PHARMACOLOGY IN SECONDARY PREVENTION

Patients are advised about the importance of taking medication as prescribed when they leave hospital.

Beta-adrenoceptor Blocking Agents

This is a group of drugs which is very widely used and has proved to be very valuable in the treatment of coronary artery disease. A drug from this group may be prescribed at one week post-infarction and continued at the discretion of the consultant in charge of the patient. A number of studies have suggested a reduction of both sudden death and re-infarction in patients taking these drugs.

Antiarrhythmic Therapy

Antiarrhythmic drugs are not prescribed for all patients who have sustained myocardial infarction. It is accepted that the majority of patients who die suddenly do so from an arrhythmia. While it is possible to identify those at high risk, it has proved difficult to identify those who will benefit from antiarrhymic drugs. Patients who have had recurrent arrhythmias while in hospital will receive appropriate medication on discharge.

Anticoaguiants

Over the years, there have been many studies into the benefits of anticoagulation after myocardial infarction. The issue remains a controversial one; some authorities believe long-term anticoagulants prevent further myocardial infarction and pulmonary and systemic embolism. In hospital, heparin and warfarin may be prescribed for those with known vascular disease, those who develop emboli, atrial fibrillation and those who are likely to require prolonged bed rest. Recent evidence has suggested that heparin may prevent infarction in patients admitted with angina. Whether anticoagulation is continued after discharge will depend on the cardiologist.

Other Drugs

Research is at present going on into drugs which reduce infarct size, e.g. hyaluronidasc. Currently thcsc havc limitcd clinical usc but they may play a big part in the future management of patients with myocardial infarction (Chapter 16).

CARDIOVASCULAR SURGERY

Coronary artery bypass surgery and angioplasty have played an important part in rehabilitation and secondary prevention over the years. Intractable chest pain caused by severe coronary artery disease can often be relieved with cardiovascular surgery. Surgery is now more common for repair of ventricular septal defects and papillary muscle dysfunction. Surgery also has an increasingly important role in the management of refractory ventricular arrhythmias (see Chapter 16).

Further Reading

Editorial. (1975). Cardiac Rehabilitation. *Journal of the Royal College of Physicians*. **9(4)**:281–346.

Holmes S. (1983). You are what you eat. *Nursing Times;* **79 (48)**:8–10.

Kellerman J.J. (1982). Comprehensive Cardiac Rehabilitation. *Advances in Cardiology*; **31**.

Norris R.M. (1982). *Myocardial infarction*, pp.102–210. Edinburgh: Churchill Livingstone.

Pedersen T.R. (1983). The Norwegian Multicenter Study of Timolol after Myocardial Infarction. *Circulation Part 11;* **67 (6)**:149–153.

Salonen J.T., Puska P. (1980). A community programme for rehabilitation and secondary prevention for patients with acute myocardial infarction as part of a comprehensive community programme for control of cardiovascular diseases (North Karelia project). *Scandanavian Journal of Rehabilitation Medicine;* **12(1)**:33–42.

Sleight P. (1982). Beta-blockade in acute myocardial infarction. In *Comprehensive Cardiac Rehabilitation. Advances in Cardiology*; **31**:90–94.

Townsend A. (1983). Endocardial resection. *Nursing Times;* **79 (43)**:64–66.

WHO Expert Committee (1964). *Rehabilitation of patients with cardiovascular diseases*. Technical Report Series No.270. p.287. Geneva: World Health Organisation.

WHO Expert Committee (1982). *Prevention of Coronary Heart Disease*. Technical report series No. 687. p.287. Geneva: World Health Organisation.

11

The Intra Aortic Balloon Pump

The intra aortic balloon pump (IABP) provides mechanical circulatory assistance to the failing heart. This is achieved by the insertion of a balloon-tipped catheter into the aorta. The balloon is inflated by the pump thus increasing the blood flow to the coronary arteries and enabling more oxygen to reach the myocardium. This technique is sometimes referred to as counterpulsation and is used when conventional methods of treatment have failed and the patient's life is in danger.

Early experimental work on this technique was carried out on animals by Kantrowitz in 1953. Later, successful work was carried out by Clauss *et al.* in 1961, and the following year Moulopoulos *et al.* published their results from work using the balloon catheter. Experimental work continued and the balloon pump of today is used to support patients over the critical part of their illness.

Indications

The IABP may be used to help children and adults during the post-operative period following cardiac surgery until the left ventricle has become more efficient. It can be used for patients in cardiogenic shock due to pump failure following myocardial infarction, but this is of limited value only as these patients usually deteriorate once the support has been withdrawn. However, if shock is associated with complications of myocardial infarction

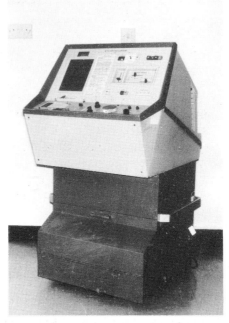

Fig. 11.1 AVCO 10 system.

such as papillary muscle dysfunction or ventricular septal defect, the IABP can be used to stabilise the situation until the role of surgery has been evaluated. Patients with unstable angina and those with resistant ventricular arrhythmias due to ischaemia also benefit from counterpulsation by improvement in the coronary artery flow. In such patients coronary angiography can then be safely undertaken.

The full list of indications is seen in Table 11.1.

Contraindications

The IABP is not used if the following exist:

1. an incompetent aortic valve.
2. a dissecting aortic aneurysm.
3. any terminal illness.

DESCRIPTION OF SYSTEMS

In the United Kingdom several intra aortic balloon pump systems are available. The AVCO systems use helium gas for inflation and

TABLE 11.1
Indications for use of the IABP

1. Unstable angina, including post infarction angina which is resistant to conventional therapy.
2. Low output state/shock due to mechanical complications of myocardial infarction, such as:
     a. ventricular septal defect,
     b. mitral regurgitation due to papillary muscle dysfunction,
     c. ventricular aneurysm.
3. Resistant ischaemic ventricular arrhythmias.
4. Cardiogenic shock due to pump failure (limited use only).
5. Low output state after cardiac surgery.

it is the AVCO 10 system which is referred to in this chapter (Fig. 11.1). The Hoek Loos model, the Charing Cross model and the Data Scope systems use carbon dioxide (Fig. 11.2). The balloons

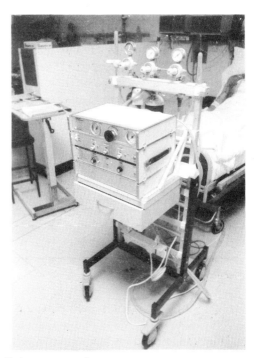

Fig. 11.2   Datascope system.

used with the AVCO model are available in various sizes from 10–40 cc, but a 4 cc paediatric size is also available. The balloon consists of a polyurethane coated catheter with non-thrombogenic properties. It is trisegmented and inflates initially from the centre, followed by inflation of the proximal and distal ends simultaneously.

The console contains the signal processing, timing and control mechanisms. It incorporates a colourful display of the patient's arterial wave-form, balloon activity and ECG, as well as a digital display of the heart rate and blood pressure (Fig. 11.3). The oscilloscope can display pre-programmed messages if there is malfunction of the machine, thereby allowing easy identification of the problem.

INSERTION OF IABP

The insertion of the balloon can be done by one of two techniques.

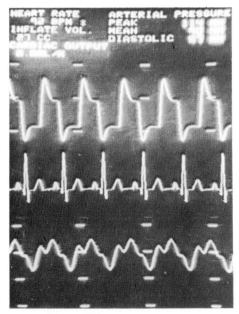

Fig. 11.3   AVCP IABP Model 10 display unit.

In the coronary care unit, the balloon can be inserted by surgical cutdown or the percutaneous approach. Both are done under strict asepsis. Occasionally the abdominal aorta is used if the femoral approach is not acceptable and this is always carried out in the theatre.

The Surgical Cutdown

This is usually performed by cutdown into the femoral artery. Once the artery is exposed, snugger clips are applied to stem the blood flow. A purse string suture is inserted into the artery and an incision made. The balloon is passed into the artery and advanced into the descending aorta to a point distal to the left subclavian artery. Sometimes a Dacron graft is sewn to the arteriotomy. The

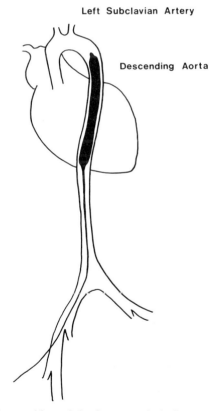

Fig. 11.4   The position of the intra aortic balloon pump (IABP).

wound is then closed and dressed. An x-ray will confirm the position of the balloon (Fig. 11.4). A separate arterial line is necessary for pressure monitoring.

Percutaneous Approach

Until 1979 the insertion of the balloon was always a surgical procedure. In this year the percutaneous balloon was adopted and this eliminated the need for surgical cutdown. This is the method more commonly used in the coronary care unit. The balloon is introduced into the femoral artery using the percutaneous Seldinger method. The balloon is wrapped tightly around the catheter and then inserted through the sheath, its position being checked by x-ray screening. Once in position the balloon is unwrapped by rotation of the catheter and it is then connected to the pump allowing inflation to begin. One advantage of the percutaneous balloon is its central lumen which allows monitoring of the arterial pressure without necessity for a separate arterial line.

TIMING

The balloon is timed to inflate in diastole and deflate in systole. This can be determined by the patient's ECG or arterial waveform. The dicrotic notch on the arterial waveform is the point at which the aortic valve closes and the balloon is set to inflate at this

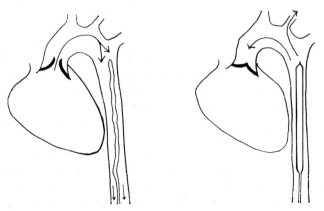

Fig. 11.5 Deflation and inflation of the IABP. Left — deflation of balloon in systole. Right — inflation of balloon in diastole.

time. Similarly diastolic inflation can be timed from the R wave on the ECG. By inflating in diastole, there is an increase in diastolic pressure in the aorta which results in a marked increase in coronary artery flow.

Deflation will occur at a preset interval or will be triggered by the next R wave. This is a safety mechanism to prevent the ventricle ejecting while the balloon is still inflated, for example, in the presence of atrial fibrillation or extrasystoles. Deflation results in decreasing afterload by up to 40% thus reducing myocardial oxygen consumption.

Inflation and deflation occurring after each cardiac cycle is known as a 1:1 ratio. When inflation and deflation occur after every second cardiac cycle, it is referred to as a 1:2 ratio.

THE NURSING CARE

The care of the patient with intra aortic balloon pump support demands not only experienced nursing but someone who can combine the understanding of advanced technology with that role. The teaching programme should therefore include counterpulsation and pressure monitoring, ensuring the nurse's confident and relaxed manner.

The patient must sign written consent for IABP insertion as this is an invasive procedure. The groin area is shaved prior to insertion. The procedure is normally done under local anaesthetic, but diamorphine hydrochloride 5 mg with prochlorperazine 12·5 mg may be given for sedation.

The patient is nursed in the position most comfortable to him. Although the ideal position is at an angle of no more than 45°, this is not always practical for a conscious patient in the CCU. He is encouraged to relax as long as he avoids undue flexion at the groin where the balloon catheter has been inserted.

Sometimes complications arise following insertion of the balloon catheter (Table 11.2). These may be a direct or indirect result of the IABP. It is important, therefore, for the nurse to carry out observations — half hourly initially and then gradually less often (Table 11.3). The care of the patient is the same as for any patient in the coronary care unit. Daily bed baths and regular pressure care are carried out. Oral toilet is given as necessary. Diet is unrestricted unless a special diet is required.

TABLE 11.2

Complications which may occur in patients with IABP

---

1. Ischaemia of the limb due to spasm, occlusion or thrombosis.
2. Infection:
   - a. at insertion site of IABP.
   - b. site of arterial line.
   - c. site of Swan Ganz catheter if inserted.
   - d. urinary catheter if inserted.
3. Haemorrhage:
   - a. at insertion of IABP.
   - b. arterial site.
4. Perforation:
   - a. femoral.
   - b. aortic.
5. Complications of bed rest.
6. Psychological complications.

The physiotherapist visits daily and basic routine exercises are carried out. The patient's wound sites are dressed aseptically and swabs are sent for culture and sensitivity as the prevention and detection of infection is of great importance in patients who may be going for cardiac surgery.

If there are no medical indications for a urinary catheter, patients can usually cope well with urinals and bedpans. It is essential to prevent constipation. Patients in cardiogenic shock will require inotropic drugs. These must be given through a central venous line. All patients with IABP support are given intravenous heparin to prevent thrombosis formation on the balloon and subsequent arterial emboli. The heparin is infused by means of digital pumps. In CCU, patients with IABP have daily urea and electrolytes and creatine phosphokinase levels taken. Before angiography and surgery, blood is taken for hepatitis B antigen and cross matching; ideally these are done at the time of balloon insertion.

Psychological Care

Nursing of the patient on an IABP requires understanding of the

TABLE 11.3
Observations required for patients with an IABP

Observations
Arterial pressure ⎫ from oscilloscope.
Heart rate   ⎭

Pulse check
Feet — dorsalis pedis.

Temperature
Warmth and colour of feet for comparison.
Core temperature.

Sites for bleeding
Arterial cannula.
Site of balloon insertion.

Check settings
1. Ratio
2. IABP on manual or automatic.

Fluid
Intake and output.

patient's fears and those of his relatives. The patient has now become more dependent for all his needs on those who are caring for him.

The nurse can do much to alleviate anxiety by simple explanations, not only of the balloon itself but of forthcoming angiography and surgery. Although both the cardiologist and surgeon will discuss the management with the patient, it is the nurse who can provide the day to day reassurance.

Removal of IABP

The length of time a balloon is left in position depends on the patient's needs. As the patient becomes less dependent on the balloon, the weaning process takes place. The ratio of the balloon is reduced to 1:2, 1:4 and then 1:8. If the balloon has been inserted as a surgical procedure, the cardiothoracic surgeon will remove it. A balloon inserted by the percutaneous approach will require removal of the balloon and sheath together, applying pressure over the femoral artery until haemostasis occurs. Regular observation of the wound is made for evidence of bleeding or infection.

Further Reading

Chrzanowski A.L. (1978). Intra aortic balloon pumping: concepts and patient care. *Nursing Clinics of North America;* **13** (3):513–530.

Clauss R.H., Birtwell W.C., Albertal G. *et al.* (1961). Assisted circulation. *Journal of Thoracic and Cardiovascular Surgery;* **41** (4):447–458.

Moulopoulos S.D., Topaz S., Kolff W.J. (1962). Diastolic balloon pumping (with carbon dioxide) in the aorta — a mechanical assistance to failing circulation. *American Heart Journal;* **63** (5):669–675.

Townsend A. (1983). The intra aortic balloon pump in the coronary care unit. *Nursing Times;* **79** (13):24–26.

12

The Pulmonary Artery Flotation Catheter

THE PULMONARY ARTERY CATHETER

The pulmonary artery (PA) flotation catheter was first introduced into clinical practice in 1970 by H.J.C. Swan and W. Ganz (Swan and Ganz, 1970). It is now frequently used as an aid to medical diagnosis and treatment.

Right heart catheterisation was described as early as 1905 by Fritz Bleichroeder and again in 1929 by Werner Forssman (Hathaway, 1978). Indeed, Forssman used a cutdown in his left antecubital vein to perform right atrial catheterisation on himself.

Over the next few decades, many developments in medical knowledge and technology took place. In 1953 balloon-tipped catheters were described by M. Lategola and H. Rahn (Lategola and Rahn, 1953) and in 1964 PA catheterisation, which could be performed at the bedside, was described by R.D. Bradley (Bradley, 1964).

Swan and Ganz perfected the balloon-tipped PA catheter and such catheters, although produced by many manufacturers, are almost universally known as Swan-Ganz catheters.

The PA Balloon-tipped Catheter — What is it?

The PA balloon-tipped catheter is a thin flexible radio-opaque tube. The small inflatable balloon near its tip allows it to float from

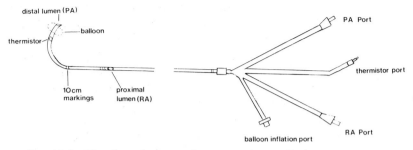

Fig. 12.1   The three lumen pulmonary artery catheter.

the right atrium into the right ventricle and onwards into the pulmonary artery.

The catheter may have two or three lumens (Fig. 12.1). The most simple two lumen type has a large lumen terminating in an opening at the catheter tip and a second smaller lumen for inflation of the balloon. The three lumen catheter has an additional proximal lumen terminating approximately 30 cm from the tip which lies in the RA when the catheter is in place. A more expensive catheter incorporates a temperature probe (thermistor) terminating approximately four centimetres from the distal tip. This catheter can be used to calculate cardiac output, using the following technique. A small volume of cold fluid is injected through the lumen leading to the RA. The thermistor records the change in temperature of the blood in the PA. From these measurements the cardiac output can be derived. This is known as the thermodilution technique.

Insertion of the PA Catheter

The PA catheter is inserted, using aseptic technique, through the jugular, subclavian, antecubital or femoral veins. The insertion site is shaved, cleaned and infiltrated with local anaesthetic. Two approaches can be used: a percutaneous approach using a Seldinger technique or a direct approach using a cutdown procedure. The catheter is passed through the peripheral vein with the balloon deflated. When the RA is entered, as evident from the pressure waveform or the position on x-ray screening, the catheter balloon is inflated with 1·5 cc of air. The catheter should then float with the blood flow through the tricuspid valve, into the right ventricle and on into the PA. The inflated balloon protects the endocardium and blood vessels from injury by the catheter tip. Eventually, the balloon lodges in one of the smaller distal branches of either the right or left pulmonary artery. This is described as the 'wedge' position, and from here, pulmonary capillary wedge pressures (PCWP) are measured. After initial measurements are recorded, the balloon is deflated. Balloon inflation times are thereafter kept to a minimum as prolonged inflation may result in necrosis of the vessel wall. X-ray screening during the procedure is helpful but not essential, as the pressure waveform gives a good indication of the catheter position. The main chambers and vessels of the heart give characteristic pressure traces which are easily recognisable on a bedside oscilloscope (Fig. 12.2). However, at the end of the insertion procedure, a chest x-ray is usually performed to confirm the position of the catheter tip, and if the subclavian approach is used, to exclude pneumothorax. The catheter is sutured in position and a sterile dressing is applied over the insertion site.

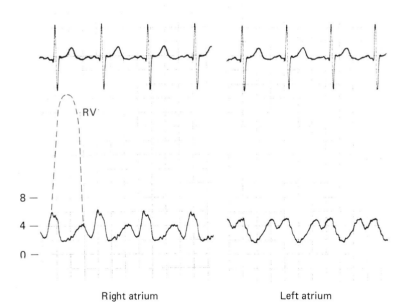

Right atrium   Left atrium

Fig. 12.2a   Pressure wave forms.

Pressure Recording

Continuous measurements from the PA can be recorded, after

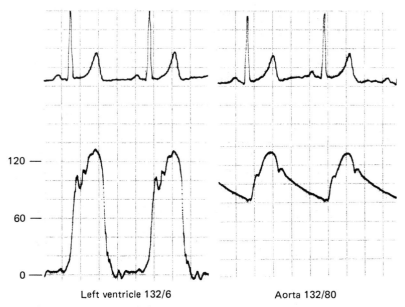

120 —

60 —

0 —

Left ventricle 132/6   Aorta 132/80

Fig. 12.2b Pressure wave forms.

insertion of the catheter. The pressures are transmitted and displayed in both wave and digital forms on a bedside oscilloscope.

The PA and RA lumens are attached by manometer lines to transducers set on a stand beside the bed. The transducers contain pressure sensitive domes which convert the pressures to the wave and digital displays. Pressures from the PA are relayed via the distal catheter lumen and RA pressures via the proximal lumen.

A continuous infusion of heparinised dextrose or saline from a pressure bag maintains the patency of the catheter and pressure lines. 'Intraflow' systems are often used to deliver fluid through the lines at a constant rate of approximately 3 ml per hour. This system also allows for more rapid flushing if required.

What is PCWP?

Pulmonary capillary wedge pressure is the pressure recorded with the balloon inflated and the catheter wedged in one of the distal branches of the PA. The inflated balloon prevents blood flow from the right side of the heart from influencing the pressures recorded. During ventricular diastole, the mitral valve is open. Thus the PCWP should be a direct reflection of the left atrial and left ventricular end diastolic pressure (LVEDP), i.e. the pressure in

TABLE 12.1
Normal intracardiac pressures (mmHg)

Right atrium	Mean	0 – 6
Right ventricle	Systolic	15 – 30
	Diastolic	0 – 5
Pulmonary artery	Systolic	15 – 30
	Diastolic	5 – 15
Pulmonary capillary wedge pressure	Mean	6 – 12
Left atrium	Mean	6 – 12
Left ventricle	Systolic	90 – 110
	Diastolic	6 – 12
Aorta	Systolic	90 – 140
	Diastolic	60 – 90

the left ventricle just before contraction. Should PCWP be difficult to obtain, PA diastolic pressure may be recorded, as the two
closely resemble each other if lung function is normal. The PA
diastolic pressure is usually slightly higher than PCWP by 1 or
2 mmHg (Table 12.1). Generally speaking, left ventricular failure
results in high PCWP; hypovolaemia results in low PCWP. If
mitral valve disease or lung disease is present, PA pressures no
longer reflect LVEDP accurately.

Indications for Measuring PCWP

Measuring PCWP is a relatively uncomplicated method of assessing left atrial pressure and left ventricular function. In previous
years, central venous pressure was used as one of the main
indicators of cardiac function. Although this is a useful measure of
right ventricular failure and circulating fluid volume, it is not
always a reliable measure of left heart function. Thus, the opportunity to measure accurate left and right ventricular function by
the insertion of one PA catheter has gained popularity.

Some indications for the use of such catheters are outlined in
Table 12.2. The PA catheter has further advantages in that it can
be used for blood sampling for oxygen saturation estimation and as
a central line through which fluids, which may cause damage to
more peripheral veins, can be infused.

TABLE 12.2
Indications for the use of the PA flotation catheter in the coronary care unit.

---

1. Diagnosis and evaluation of:
    Cardiogenic shock
    Hypovolaemia
    Pulmonary oedema
    Ventricular septal defect post myocardial infarction
    Mitral regurgitation post myocardial infarction.
2. Monitoring of therapy in critically ill patients.

NURSING RESPONSIBILITIES

The nurse has an important role to play before, during and after insertion of a PA catheter. Her initial responsibilities include the psychological preparation of the patient with simple, clear explanations of the procedure and reassurance that it should not be painful. It is also important that the patient's relatives are informed of what is happening. Similar explanations of the procedure and what to expect afterward should be given to them.

Physical preparation of the patient includes shaving the insertion site, ensuring he is not allergic to the iodine-based skin cleaning solution, and dressing him appropriately. A consent form should be signed by the patient. The procedure room has to be prepared and the necessary equipment assembled; the resuscitation trolley must be near at hand. X-ray technicians may need to be alerted to screen the procedure; physiological measurement technicians are available in some hospitals to organise the technical setting up of the transducer and flush systems and to calibrate the equipment. In other centres, this is carried out by the medical or nursing staff. During the procedure, the nurse's responsibilities include reassuring the patient, assisting the doctor and observing the monitors closely for evidence of ectopic beats or more sustained arrhythmias.

After the PA catheter has been inserted, the nurse's responsibilities fall into three categories:

1. technical care of the equipment.

2. physical care of the patient.
3. psychological care of the patient and his relatives.

Technical Care of the Equipment

The transducer set up must be well maintained if accurate PA and RA measurements are to be recorded.

Reference point

To obtain accurate pressures and to eliminate errors due to spontaneous changes in position, it is essential that the transducers are always placed at a constant reference point in relation to the patient's body before each recording is made. The patient is usually asked to lie on his back in a semi-recumbent position and a point in the fourth intercostal space in the axillary line is used as the reference point.

Calibration

Before measurements are recorded, the transducers should be tested to ensure that they are working accurately. They should record zero when exposed to atmospheric pressure and in some systems can be tested against a column of water at a known height, e.g. if a transducer is exposed to a column of water measuring 50 cm, the digital display should record 50. When it is then exposed to the pressures within the patient's body, it should record these accurately.

Recording PCWP

PCWP may be recorded intermittently by inflating the catheter balloon thus wedging it in one of the branches of the PA. In some hospitals, the medical staff prefer to record these measurements. They should never be recorded by anyone who does not understand the dangers of over-inflation or prolonged inflation of the balloon.

Observations

Routine observations of blood pressure, heart rate and rhythm, respiratory rate and temperature are made in addition to regular PA and RA pressure recordings. Nursing and medical staff must be familiar with normal intracardiac pressures and waveforms. Alteration of the PA waveform trace may indicate that the tip of the catheter has moved into a wedge position, or slipped back into the right ventricle. Damped tracings may also suggest that the catheter has become kinked or blocked. Reporting of changes to the senior nurse on duty is vital.

Physical Care of the Patient

The physical care required by a patient with a PA catheter in position is similar to that of any patient who is confined to bed and has an intravenous infusion in progress. The insertion site must be carefully observed for signs of infection, bleeding or thrombophlebitis. The sterile dressing should be changed as often as required for the patient's comfort. If additional intravenous or arterial lines are present, their patency and insertion sites must be cared for in the same way. Swabs may be sent from the sites for culture and sensitivity, and antibiotics prescribed if there is infection. Other medication is given as prescribed by the medical staff. General hygiene must be meticulous; a daily bed bath and regular care of pressure areas, mouth and hair is important. Usually the patient may eat and drink what he wants, although there may be restrictions on occasions. The patient's fluid balance is always recorded.

Sometimes a urinary catheter is inserted, so catheter care is necessary. Alternatively, when a urine bottle or bedpan is used, care must be taken not to dislodge the PA line. Aperients may be required to prevent constipation. Regular movement in bed and physiotherapy is encouraged to prevent such complications of bed rest as infections and deep venous thrombosis.

Psychological Care of the Patient and his Relatives

The importance of good psychological care of the patient and his relatives cannot be overemphasised. Simple unhurried explanations will go a long way to reassure them and gain their cooperation. Time must be found to give information and to update it frequently.

Removal

Ideally the PA catheter should be removed after approximately 48 hours, although sometimes the patient's condition dictates that it remain in place for longer periods. Its removal is an aseptic procedure. After a simple explanation to the patient, a check is made to make sure the balloon is deflated. The suture is removed and the catheter is gently withdrawn. The patient's cardiac rhythm is closely observed for arrhythmias during the procedure. A sterile dressing is applied to the site.

In view of the cost of PA catheters, there is a temptation to resterilise and reuse them. This is not recommended by the manufacturers and attention has been drawn to the problem of clot formation on reused catheters.

COMPLICATIONS

Although the use of PA catheters for haemodynamic monitoring is thought to be relatively safe, there are several possible complications of which the staff must be aware. Pneumothorax, emboli and the introduction of infection are possible problems with the insertion procedure. Infection may occur at the site or may, on rare occasions, result in endocarditis or septicaemia. Occasionally the catheter becomes kinked or coiled during insertion. Should this occur, the balloon is deflated, and the catheter is withdrawn and straightened before being reinserted.

Arrhythmias are not uncommon, particularly while the catheter is being floated onwards through the heart valves and chambers. They often take the form of atrial or ventricular ectopics but emergency equipment is always available in case more dangerous ectopic rhythms arise. Ventricular arrhythmias may also result from the catheter slipping from its position in the pulmonary artery back into the right ventricle.

Perforation of the PA has been reported as a problem associated with PA catheters. Pulmonary infarction may result from prolonged inflation of the balloon or movement of the catheter further into the artery to block a distal branch. Air embolism is sometimes a complication of the PA catheter if the balloon is burst following its inflation. Thromboembolism may also occur as a result of emboli forming on the tip of the catheter and then becoming dislodged.

The more experienced the doctors and nurses carrying out the procedure, the less likely are complications to arise.

References

Bradley R.D. (1964). Diagnostic right-heart catheterisation with miniature catheters in severely ill patients. *Lancet;* **2**:941–942.

Hathaway R. (1978). The Swan–Ganz Catheter: a Review. *Nursing Clinics of North America;* **13**:389–407.

Lategola M., Rahn H. (1953). A self-guiding catheter for cardiac and pulmonary arterial catheterisation and occlusion. *Proceedings of the Society of Experimental Biological Sciences;* **84**:667–668.

Swan H.J.C., Ganz W., Forrester J., *et al.* (1970). Catheterisation of the heart in men with use of a flow-directed balloon-tipped catheter. *New England Journal of Medicine;* **283**:447–451.

Further Reading

Andreoli K.G., Hunn–Fowkes V., Zipes D.P., Wallace A.G. (1979). *Comprehensive Cardiac Care: a Text for Nurses, Physicians and Other Health Practitioners*, 4th edn., pp.79–82 and 287–290. St. Louis: The C.V. Mosby Company.

Applefeld J.J., Caruthers T.E., Reno D.J., Civetta J.M. (1978). Assessment of the Sterility of Long-Term Cardiac Catheterisation Using the Thermodilution Swan–Ganz Catheter. *Chest;* **74**:377–380.

George R.J.D., Banks R.A. (1983). Bedside measurement of pulmonary capillary wedge pressure. *British Journal of Hospital Medicine;* **29**:286–291.

Lalli S.M. (1978). The complete Swan–Ganz. *Registered Nurse;* **41**:64–77.

McCulloch J. (1983). The Pulmonary Artery Catheter. *Nursing Times;* **79**:27–30.

Woods S.L. (1976). Monitoring Pulmonary Artery Pressures. *The American Journal of Nursing;* **76**:1765–1771.

13

Other Disorders Seen in Coronary Care Units

Staff working on Coronary Care Units should be constantly alert to the possibility of other acute medical conditions masquerading as angina and myocardial infarction. Inevitably many patients accepted for acute admission will be found not to have a cardiac problem. Some hospitals evaluate all potential admissions in a receiving area before transfer to the CCU, others prefer to undertake the initial evaluation on the CCU itself. Whichever policy is adopted, it is important that all acute coronary care facilities are immediately available to the patient wherever he is seen first.

If the diagnosis is uncertain, patients may be retained on the CCU until a series of ECGs and initial enzymes are obtained. The size of the CCU and bed availability will determine how soon such patients will be transferred to a ward situation. It should always be remembered that the first indication of an impending infarction may be vague chest pain with a normal examination and ECG. Occasionally such patients, apparently stable on admission, may infarct after their transfer to the ward. In some situations, this may be unavoidable, so ideally the ward to which they are transferred should be close to the CCU. All patients should, if possible, have a firm diagnosis established before transfer. They can then be moved to an appropriate area, for example, a general surgical ward or thoracic medical ward. Those without an established diagnosis will require further investigation and are best moved to the ward for post-infarction patients. The smooth efficiency of a CCU involved in frequent admissions and discharges demands the close cooperation of other medical and nursing staff throughout the hospital.

The range of medical problems electively nursed on a CCU will be determined by many factors, some of which will depend on the other facilities available in the individual hospital. Where an ITU and CCU are separate, clear policy guidelines are required. Although the training of nursing staff allows them to work effectively in either situation, the emphasis of the units is different; although there is much overlap between the two, anaesthetists tend to direct ITUs and physicians manage the CCUs. Acute conditions requiring mechanical ventilation are usually therefore treated in the ITU and problems such as arrhythmias in the CCU. Frequently these problems coexist and the best environment for such a patient will require careful consideration. A close working relationship between these units is important and the expertise within them should always be available to the other.

A CCU provides not only intensive care, but also the facilities for intensive observation. If a clinical problem requires close observation for either diagnostic or therapeutic purposes, it may be better dealt with on a CCU even if ischaemic heart disease is not suspected. This again will be determined by the facilities on the general ward and particularly the number of staff available; the value of a bedside monitor for detecting temporary rhythm disturbances on a ward is of limited value if the staff are too busy and not available to observe it.

The non-ischaemic problems encountered on a CCU, either arriving 'by accident' or electively admitted, are many and varied. Coronary care staff working in this area over a period of time will encounter a wide range of medical and cardiological conditions. Some of these are considered below.

Sick Sinus Syndrome

In this condition, the automatic pacemaker function of the sinus node is depressed. The underlying pathology is usually degenerative and therefore the condition is more common in the elderly. This depression may be permanent or intermittent and may result in sinus bradycardia or episodes of asystole occurring during apparently normal rhythm. Many patients will present with a history of episodic dizziness or syncope and the underlying cause may not be immediately apparent unless a recording is taken at the time of symptoms. Frequently such patients also exhibit paroxysms of supraventricular tachycardia, a conditon known as the 'brady–tachy' syndrome, and this may be the first presentation of a sick sinus problem.

There may be a number of clues to the nature of the underlying condition. When the bradycardia occurs, it will tend to be inappropriate to the clinical situation. The normal sinus tachycardia response to stress and exercise is often reduced and the rate response to atropine may be blunted. With a normal heart rate, there may be exaggerated slowing with carotid sinus massage. Important observations may be made during the tachycardia phase. At the moment of termination, there may be a prolonged period of sinus arrest before the normal pacemaker recovers. This may be observed with spontaneous termination, but also after DC cardioversion and drug treatment. Drugs that suppress tachycardias and tend to slow the heart rate, for example, beta-adrenoceptor blocking agents, may induce profound bradycardia and asystole in patients with the sick sinus syndrome.

Long-term pacing should abolish the symptoms due to bradycardia, but drugs may be required in addition to control the associated tachycardia. With a pacemaker implanted, these drugs can be used more freely without the fear of bradycardia.

The Wolff–Parkinson–White (WPW) Syndrome

Normally the atria are electrically insulated from the ventricles apart from a small area containing the AV node through which the sinus impulses pass to activate the ventricles. Patients with this syndrome (WPW) have an additional or accessory conducting pathway which connects the atria to the ventricles, allowing some of the electrical impulses to bypass the junctional tissue. Under these circumstances, the ventricles are depolarised from two sources. Since the accessory pathway does not slow the impulse in the same way as the AV node, the part of the ventricle close to the insertion of pathway is depolarised first (pre-excitation). This produces the characteristic slurred delta wave at the start of QRS. Since propagation of the impulse from the pathway through the myocardium is slow, the contribution through the AV node and the bundle branches rapidly catches up and overtakes to produce the normal terminal part of the QRS. The total QRS complex is, therefore, a fusion of depolarisation from these two sources (Fig. 13.1.).

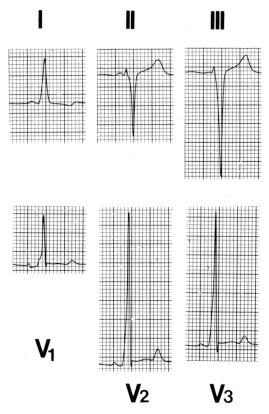

Fig. 13.1   The ECG of a patient with the Wolff–Parkinson–White syndrome.

If the impulses from the atria always split to take both parallel routes to the ventricle, the syndrome would be no more than an electrocardiographic curiosity. However, if the impulses only take one antegrade route, the other become immediately available to conduct retrogradely. Thus the ideal scene is set for a re-entry mechanism (Fig. 13.2.). Clinically, supraventricular tachycardias due to this cause can be a considerable problem in some patients with this syndrome. Occasionally the pathway cannot conduct in an antegrade manner and is said to be concealed since the characteristic delta wave is not produced and the QRS complexes are normal. Nevertheless, retrograde conduction through the pathway can still occur and induce a re-entry tachycardia.

AVR   AVL   AVF

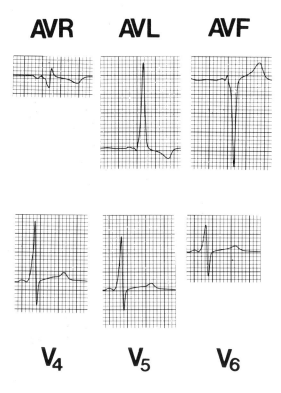

V₄   V₅   V₆

Fig. 13.1   Contd.

Because conduction through the AV node is slow, it protects the ventricles against following rapid supraventricular arrhythmias. For example, many of the impulses during atrial fibrillation are blocked and never reach the ventricle. Bypass pathways usually do not have this protective effect and tend to conduct rapidly, thus producing a potentially dangerous situation. In the WPW syndrome, therefore, atrial fibrillation can produce a much faster ventricular response which may lead to serious ventricular arrhythmias. The well established higher incidence of sudden death in this syndrome is almost certainly due to rapid supraventricular rhythms inducing ventricular fibrillation through fast conducting pathways.

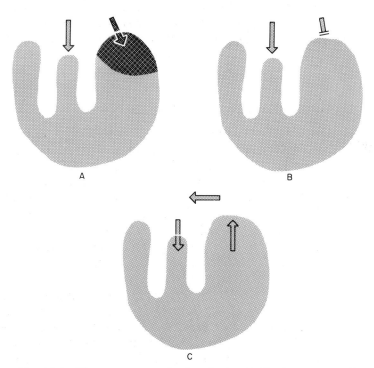

Fig. 13.2   The re-entry mechanism in the Wolff—Parkinson—White syndrome. (a) Conduction through AV node and accessory pathway. (b) Accessory pathway block. AV node conduction only. (c) Re-entry retrogradely through accessory pathway.

Successful drug treatment of the arrhythmias associated with this syndrome may be very difficult and may require detailed invasive electrophysiological studies. The anatomical position and conduction properties of the pathways can be accurately determined, and using specialised pacing techniques during these studies, often the arrhythmias can be easily started and terminated. This allows the effects of various drugs to be studied acutely and those found to be effective, identified for the future long-term oral use. It is important to appreciate that those patients at high risk can be identified during these investigations. It has become possible to identify and surgically divide these pathways and many patients, who were at risk and whose arrhythmias were refractory to drugs, have obtained lasting benefit from a surgical approach. Recent work has suggested that selective injury to some pathways can be achieved during electrophysiological studies without the necessity for cardiac surgery. If this benefit is maintained for significant periods, it will certainly widen the application of this method of treatment.

Pulmonary Embolism

In this condition, a venous thrombus which has developed usually in the legs or pelvis becomes detached from its site of origin and is carried with the flow of blood through the right heart chambers into the pulmonary artery. The size of the embolus will determine the level at which it obstructs the pulmonary artery. A small embolus may be carried into the periphery of the lung and block the blood supply to only a small portion of lung tissue, whereas a large embolus may wedge in the larger branches and deprive a much greater area of lung of its blood flow. These factors determine the way in which the condition presents clinically.

When only a small peripheral pulmonary artery is blocked, the extra work that the right ventricle has to do in pumping blood through the lung will be small and the embolism will tend to cause few or no symptoms. Symptoms that do arise, develop later and are due to the area of infarction of lung tissue that results. Thus pleuritic pain and haemoptysis are common and a pleural rub may be heard over the area of infarction. The ECG is frequently normal, but the chest x-ray may show a wedge-shaped area of shadowing, elevation of the diaphragm and a small effusion.

A large or massive pulmonary embolism presents suddenly at the time the embolism occurs. There is a major acute obstruction to blood flow through the lungs and the right ventricle is unable to cope with the extra work required to pump against this resistance. This may result in sudden collapse and death or in the clinical features of acute heart failure. Hyperventilation, tachycardia, hypotension or elevation of the jugular venous pressure may be evident. The chest x-ray is often unhelpful and only occasionally is the oligaemia, due to the reduced blood flow and less prominent pulmonary vessels, convincing. However, the ECG is often very helpful (Fig. 13.3) and will show signs of acute right ventricular strain — T wave inversion in V_1, V_2, V_3.

The classical S wave in lead 1 and the Q wave and T inversion in

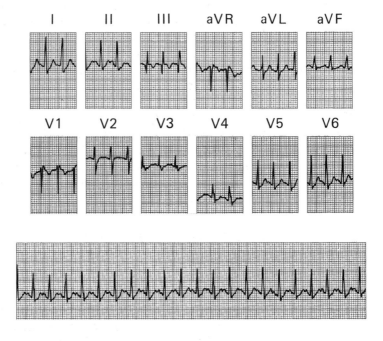

Fig. 13.3   The ECG of a patient with an acute pulmonary embolus showing an S wave in lead I, a Q wave and an inverted T wave in lead III, and partial right bundle branch block.

lead III reflect this strain and the change in electrical axis that results from it. There are, of course, varying degrees of severity of pulmonary embolism and the features may vary between these two extremes described. Radio-isotope lung scans have proved to be most helpful in detecting areas of reduced pulmonary blood flow and confirming the diagnosis when it is in doubt.

Whenever possible, attempts should be made to identify patients at risk and preventative measures adopted to minimise the likelihood of venous stasis and thrombosis. Prolonged immobilisation, particularly after surgery and child birth, should be avoided and early mobilisation should be encouraged. When this is not possible, leg exercises and support stockings are valuable. Prophylactic anticoagulation may be desirable, especially in patients with heart failure or a previous history of venous thrombosis.

The occurrence of pulmonary embolism demands anticoagulant treatment, initially with heparin and maintained with an oral preparation, such as warfarin, for about 6–8 weeks. If the embolism is severe and life-threatening, dissolution of the embolus with streptokinase is frequently recommended. Since this has potential dangers, it is preferable to confirm the diagnosis and evaluate its severity by right heart catheterisation and pulmonary angiography. The catheter may be left in the pulmonary artery to infuse the drug and allow constant evaluation of changes in pulmonary arterial pressure. Repeat angiography using the same catheter after a period of treatment permits the effects to be accurately determined. Such patients require intensive nursing and close observation and are frequently managed on CCUs.

Dissecting Aneurysm of the Aorta

Between the inner layer (intima) and outer layer (adventitia) of the wall of the aorta, lies a potential space occupied by the media. If the media is softened and degenerative, as occurs in Marfan's Syndrome and occasionally in pregnancy, an injury or tear in the intima may allow blood to enter the media and dissect along the length of the vessel. This will create a 'double-barrel shotgun effect' with two lumens — the true or natural lumen of the aorta and the false lumen created by the blood dissecting along the media. This condition frequently presents with severe searing chest pain and may be extremely difficult in the early stages to distinguish from an acute myocardial infarction. As many of these patients are admitted to the CCU, the staff should be aware of this condition.

The onset is often precipitated by exertion, particularly in hypertensive patients with atherosclerosis. The clinical features will depend on the site of the initial tear or entry point and whether the blood dissects proximally along the aorta towards the heart or distally. Involvement of the ascending aorta may extend to the aortic valve and produce aortic regurgitation. Frequently branches of the aorta are involved and compressed and the many different presentations reflect which vessels are affected. Thus ischaemia due to involvement of a carotid artery may cause hemiplegia, whereas a coronary artery will produce myocardial infarction and a subclavian artery will result in an ischaemic arm. All the branches of the aorta can potentially be involved.

The blood in the false lumen may do one of three things. It may re-enter the true lumen through the intima at a point further down the aorta. It may remain within the wall ultimately clotting and obliterating the space it has created. The most dangerous complication would be for it to rupture through the adventitia externally; then there would be extensive haemorrhage into the pericardial or pleural spaces or into the mediastinal or retroperitoneal tissues, depending on the site of rupture.

Although many patients will appear shocked and in severe pain, the blood pressure may be normal or high. It should be regarded as a matter of urgency to lower the blood pressure to prevent the dissection from progressing. This, together with pain relief, are the essentials of medical management. Prompt control can be better achieved by the infusion of intravenous drugs and many prefer to monitor the blood pressure response by intra-arterial recordings. Although the risks of surgery are high, it may be required if the dissection continues to progress or if complications occur. Generally, conservative management is preferred for dissection involving the descending aorta whereas ascending aortic involvement, particularly involving the aortic valve, has a worse prognosis and some centres advocate urgent surgery. The extent of the dissection can be clearly demonstrated by aortography which is an essential investigation if surgery is considered.

Cardiomyopathy

This term implies a disorder of the myocardium which upsets its normal mechanical function. By definition it does not include heart disease due to coronary arteriosclerosis, hypertension, congenital lesions or rheumatic heart disease.

It may present in one of three forms:

1. Congestive cardiomyopathy, the features being those of congestive heart failure.
2. Hypertrophic cardiomyopathy, in which the bulk of myocardium is increased, but particularly that of the intraventricular septum. This often encroaches on the outflow trace of the left ventricle producing a pressure gradient and murmur (Hypertrophic Obstructive Cardiomyopathy – HOCM). Presenting features include syncope and arrhythmias and may precipitate admission to a CCU. During the latter stages of this condition, congestive features become more common.

3.   Restrictive cardiomyopathy, when the myocardium is unable
     to dilate properly in diastole and thus impedes the normal
     filling of the ventricles. Amyloidosis affecting the heart is the
     most common cause. The clinical features are very similar to
     constrictive pericarditis and differentiation may be difficult.

Cardiomyopathy may present when the heart is one of several
organs involved in connective tissue diseases such as polyarteritis
nodosa and lupus erythematosis, or the heart may appear to be
affected alone. Alcohol has emerged as an important cause and the
history should always include an evaluation of the patient's drink-
ing habits. Cardiomyopathy can present towards the end of
pregnancy or early peurperium, although it is rare. Even if
successfully treated, it is liable to recur with subsequent pregnan-
cies.

The medical treatment of congestive cardiomyopathy is no
different to that of other types of congestive heart failure. Initially
the response may be good, but the condition inevitably progresses
and the prognosis is poor. Hypertrophic cardiomyopathies, particularly those with obstructive features, may improve with beta-
adrenergic blocking drugs. Surgical removal of hypertrophic
septal tissue (myomectomy) may be indicated in severely symptomatic patients when medical treatment has failed; it is frequently successful.

14

Unit Management
by Mrs. L. Walton   Nursing Officer

The first priority of all nurses is to ensure a high standard of patient care. Additional priorities of a nurse manager include:

1. the training and development of nursing staff.
2. the maintenance of good staffing levels, to ensure that the other priorities can be carried out effectively.

The high dependency nature of CCUs usually requires a funded establishment greater than that of a ward, but less than an ICU. A nurse-patient ratio of 3:1 is sufficient, allowing the normal percentages for holidays and sickness.

The unit should be staffed by qualified nurses — Registered General Nurses (RGNs) and Enrolled Nurses (ENs) and a minimum number of auxiliary nurses. The actual numbers of the grades of qualified nurses depends upon the number of beds in the unit and local nursing policies.

A nurse trained in coronary care nursing should have a thorough knowledge of cardiac disease and the associated problems. She must be aware of the nursing care likely to be required by her patients and she must be an expert in the specialised techniques discussed and described in this book.

Recruitment and Selection of Staff

Recruitment is usually by means of a local bulletin, local and national press, and the nursing press, although the latter would probably only be necessary for advertising senior nursing posts.

Careful selection of staff is important. The nurse must be able to cope with fluctuations in work load. She should learn to be self-reliant and she should be as efficient and effective when all is quiet and running smoothly, as she is required to be when working under stress.

Nursing Officer

The Nursing Officer responsible for the CCU should, ideally, be a trained coronary care nurse. She must have some degree of clinical involvement and she is responsible for maintaining her own expertise. She must be aware of the training and development needs of sisters and nursing staff and be able to either carry out this training or assist in its implementation. The Nursing Officer is responsible for the selection of all grades of nursing staff within the unit. Other duties include recording sickness and absence, teaching, counselling and assisting the unit sisters when requested. It is her responsibility to ensure the sisters have the facilities to fulfill their role.

CCU Staff

The unit nursing sisters are required to have a high degree of clinical knowledge and expertise. They must have a capacity for leadership and the ability to teach. Each sister should be able to delegate responsibility and allow the staff to share in decision making. She must be able to exercise authority when necessary and tolerate her staff's reaction to it. The unit sisters are also involved in the interviewing of staff and should have the right of veto.

Staff nurses and enrolled nurses are generally accepted as being a mobile population, especially in high dependency areas. Taking an objective view, the advantages of this outweigh the disadvantages. Newcomers bring fresh personalities, different ideas and possibly experience from units in other health authorities. A slow but steady turnover of staff is not only to be expected, but is also desirable. However, no one likes to lose a valued member whose abilities and personality is known to all concerned.

Auxiliary nurses are valuable members of the nursing team, although it is recommended that they be kept to a minimum number. Within the limits of their role, the auxiliary nurse can be taught to record the temperature, pulse, respiration and blood pressure of the patient. The auxiliary nurse can observe the recordings on the pressure monitor, note a change in the condition of a patient and recognise a life-threatening situation. Their instruction should stress that the only action the auxiliary nurse should take is to inform the nurse responsible for the patient or to summon help.

The National Boards — Continuing Education and Training

Many health authorities finance the National Board Continuing Education and Training Courses in coronary care nursing. These courses are available to RGNs and ENs, with separate courses for each grade. The curriculum is the same for both grades, with the exception of the research and management objectives which are taught only to RGNs.

A hospital is accepted by one of the national boards to train coronary care nurses if its facilities, expertise and commitment is of an acceptable standard. The training is regularly reviewed.

The unit sisters and the Nursing Officer are expected to teach in the classroom as well as in the practical area. The Nursing Officer — and in her absence, a sister — together with the Clinical Instructor and the Post Basic Tutor, are involved in the selection of post basic students.

Student nurses are also allocated to CCUs to gain experience in acute and high dependency nursing, usually as part of their 'trauma' module. All students, whether basic or post basic (see references), should be supernumerary to the permanent nursing staff so that the necessary supervision can be given and a learning environment can be maintained.

Teaching of Staff

Training programmes must be available for each grade of staff. The aims and objectives should be discussed with each new member and the strengths and weaknesses of the nurse identified. Each training schedule should commence with general objectives, such as introduction to staff, the geography of the unit, the siting of equipment and contents of cupboards, the patient–nurse call, the emergency call, the cardiac arrest and fire telephone numbers, the resuscitation techniques and the fire drill. The nurse also needs to be introduced to the principles of coronary care nursing and cardiac monitoring.

All grades of nursing staff can be involved in teaching, a skill often denied by the junior members of staff. The more technical aspects of care should be taught by the senior nursing staff. Senior medical staff should also be involved in the teaching of nurses and are often delighted to participate in these programmes.

Extension of the Nurse's Role

Within CCUs nurses are permitted to extend their role into areas which are normally considered a medical responsibility. All units should train nurses to administer DC shock therapy. Many are trained to give intravenous drugs via an established route and to take venous blood samples. Local policies and requirements will dictate the ways in which a nurse may extend her role; however, the nurse must always be aware of the legal implications of undertaking a role which is normally the responsibility of medical staff. Training programmes and methods of assessment must be accepted by the local Extension of the Nurse's Role Committee. The consultant in administrative charge of the unit must agree with the training given and the method of assessment of proficiency. The nurse is responsible for maintaining her proficiency in the task.

Deployment of Staff

It is the responsibility of the senior nurse on duty to allocate staff to their patients. The nurses should work in pairs, an experienced nurse with a less experienced nurse. Using a problem-solving approach, they must plan the care of the patients. The medical diagnosis and patient's condition will determine the degree and style of nursing intervention. In such an acute area, the patient and his problems should be discussed at the beginning of each span of duty. If possible, all staff on duty should attend these discussions, and nurses need to be aware that the psychological as well as the physiological condition of the patient may alter considerably during his short stay in the CCU.

Policies

Ideally, an administrative and therapeutic policy, compiled and agreed upon by all consultant medical staff involved in the care of the patients on the unit, should be available to the nursing staff. This enables the unit sister to make decisions in line with the policy while maintaining her role as a nurse.

Unit nursing policies should also be available. They must be reviewed regularly and they must be sufficiently flexible to allow the senior nurse on duty to make decisions according to the demands of any situation. These policies should be in line with the hospital and health authority.

The maintenance of supplies and equipment is an important aspect of management. A sister or senior nurse should be delegated this responsibility, thus ensuring some degree of control. In turn she can involve other members of the nursing team, allowing continuity and an increased awareness of cost.

It is the responsibility of the unit sister to ensure that her staff are familiar with fire drill. Although it is not practical to have mock fire drills, the fire officer can and should visit the unit and advise all personnel on the procedure should a fire occur.

Stress

Coronary Care Units are often considered stressful places in which to work; this is unfortunate and not necessarily correct. Certainly in areas of sophisticated technology and where there are very ill patients, many demands are made of the nurse, both physically and emotionally. Not only is the care of the patient very involved, but so too is the care of his relatives. Feeling stressed is not a weakness but rather a natural response to a stressful environment. However, much can be done and much is being done in many CCUs to alleviate the problem.

An awareness that the problem exists is the first step to dealing with it. Unit managers are careful in their selection of staff to find nurses who enjoy acute nursing, an erratic workload and a constant turnover of patients. The nurses must understand the importance of technology and invasive techniques and accept them as their aid to good patient care. In turn, senior nursing staff on CCUs must accept their responsibility to educate and support new members of staff. An efficient communication system is vital and regular opportunities for staff to meet and discuss their patients and their feelings may help to lessen the strain. Individual or group counselling sessions may also help.

It requires sustained effort and awareness on the part of nurse managers to create a relaxed and friendly atmosphere in which to work. This does not imply lack of discipline. Discipline is necessary and accepted by everyone, but the nurse who learns to discipline herself and maintain her professionalism while caring for her patients has surely achieved the ideal for which we all should strive.

Further Reading

Bishop V. (1981). This is the age of the Strain. *Nursing Mirror;* **153** (**6**):18–19.

Braun A.E. (1983). Proper staffing schedules: a must for coronary care. *Nursing Management;* **14** (**10**):27–28.

Joint Board of Clinical Nursing Studies. (1981). *Review of the Work of the Joint Board of Clinical Nursing Studies 1970–1980.* London and Reading: The Eastern Press Ltd., pp.40.

Nichols K.A., Springford V., Searle J. (1981). An investigation of distress and discontent in various types of nursing. *Journal of Advanced Nursing;* **6**: 311–318.

Rogers J., Barrett J. (1981). Choosing and using post basic clinical training. *Nursing Times;* **77** (**17**):291–293.

Roper N., Logan W., and Tierney A. (1980). *The Elements of Nursing.* Edinburgh: Churchill Livingstone.

Storlie F.J. (1979). Burnout: the elaboration of a concept. *American Journal of Nursing;* **79** (**12**):2108–2111.

Stress and Stress Management: an overview. (Including 5 articles on intensive care nurses). *Journal of Nursing Administration;* **19** (**6**):5–63.

Wilson–Barnett J. (1984). Coping with Stress. *Nursing Mirror;* **158** (**14**):16.

15

Drugs in the Coronary Care Unit

DRUGS AND THE TREATMENT OF ARRHYTHMIAS

Many drugs with anti-arrhythmic properties are now available. They possess different pharmacological properties and side-effects and the selection of a particular drug for a specific arrhythmia is not always easy. Clinical experience over many years often determines which is chosen, but more recently electrophysiological techniques have allowed a more critical evaluation of arrhythmias and drug therapy. The knowledge of how arrhythmias develop and how drugs act is fundamental to an understanding of coronary care.

Anti-arrhythmic drugs can be classified in two ways. The first is related to the electrophysiological effects on the cellular action potential and the second to the part of the heart in which these effects are chiefly seen. Although both systems are interrelated, the first can be thought of as physiological and the second as anatomical.

Physiological Classification (Vaughan Williams)

The various effects of drugs are considered in four classes according to this classification (Fig. 15.1).

Class 1
The response of the cell membrane is reduced and the transmis-

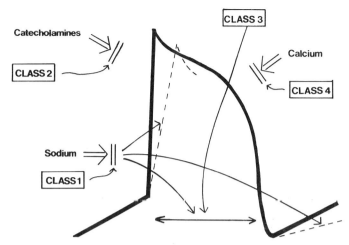

Fig. 15.1   *The physiological classification: the various effects of drugs are considered in four classes.*

sion of the impulse is slowed. The action potential shows a slower rise in Phase 0 and the spontaneous depolarisation in diastole is depressed (Phase 4). This class can be subdivided into three groups depending on what happens to the duration of the action potential. In 1A, it is prolonged; in 1B, it is shortened; and in 1C, it is not affected.

Class 2
These drugs block the effects of sympathetic stimulation but do not have a direct effect themselves on the action potential at the usual therapeutic dosage.

Class 3
These drugs prolong the action potential but without affecting its generation.

Class 4
These drugs reduce the rate of entry of calcium into the cells and depress the plateau (Phase 2, 3) of the action potential.

Table of Drug Classification

Class 1   A — quinidine, procainamide, disopyramide.
          B — lignocaine, mexiletine, phenytoin, aprindine, encainide, tocainide.
          C — flecainide.

Class 2   — beta-adrenergic blocking drugs, bretylium.
Class 3   — amiodarone, sotalol, bretylium, disopyramide.
Class 4   — verapamil.

Anatomical Classification

When an arrhythmia has been diagnosed, it should be possible to determine at which site the effect of a drug is required: for example, the atria with atrial arrhythmias, the ventricle with ventricular tachycardia, the AV node with junctional tachycardia and the bypass pathway in patients with WPW syndrome. Although some drugs have actions at more than one site, a classification of this type is clinically very useful. It has long been appreciated that the autonomic nervous system has important effects on heart rhythm so the effects of some drugs on sympathetic and parasympathetic tone should also be considered. Figure 15.2 illustrates the sites of action of many commonly used drugs and provides a useful basis for drug selection depending on the clinical situation.

Some Basic Prescribing Principles

Following myocardial infarction, the absorption of drugs from the gastrointestinal tract may be unpredictable. In addition, abnormal function of liver or kidneys may significantly affect the metabolism of the drugs given and doses may need to be adjusted.

Drugs given by constant infusion or on regular dosage schedule will take three to five times their half-life to reach steady state therapeutic levels. A half-life is defined as the time taken for a drug to fall to half its previous level. Control of arrhythmias may be urgent and to achieve a rapid therapeutic response, a loading dose will be required. This can be achieved with a high initial infusion rate or a large first oral dose. When a drug is stopped, it takes about three times its half-life for 90% to be eliminated. This should be considered when changing from one drug to another, such as discontinuing a lignocaine infusion and starting an oral preparation. Blood levels of many anti-arrhythmic drugs can be estimated and this is often useful when evaluating the adequacy of a prescribed drug regime. Although recommended schedules are appropriate for the majority of patients, there will be some exceptions. During an infusion, blood can be taken at any conve-

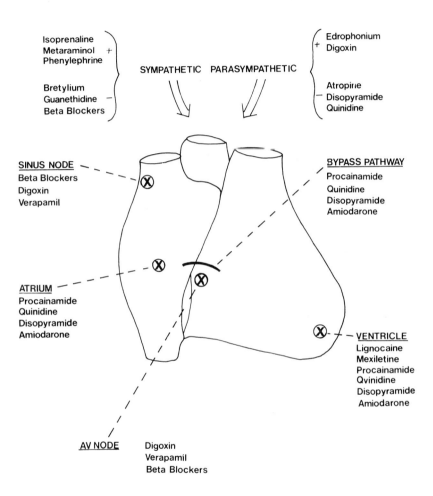

Isoprenaline
Metaraminol   +
Phenylephrine

Bretylium
Guanethidine   −
Beta Blockers

SYMPATHETIC   PARASYMPATHETIC

Edrophonium
+ Digoxin

Atropine
− Disopyramide
Quinidine

SINUS NODE
Beta Blockers
Digoxin
Verapamil

BYPASS PATHWAY
Procainamide
Quinidine
Disopyramide
Amiodarone

ATRIUM
Procainamide
Quinidine
Disopyramide
Amiodarone

VENTRICLE
Lignocaine
Mexiletine
Procainamide
Qvinidine
Disopyramide
Amiodarone

AV NODE   Digoxin
Verapamil
Beta Blockers

Fig. 15.2   The anatomical classification: this illustrates the sites of
action of many commonly used drugs and provides a useful basis for
drug selection depending on the clinical situation.

nient time provided there has been no alteration in infusion rate or concentration for 1–2 hours. When drugs are given intermittently, blood levels will vary depending upon the timing of the dose. Blood taken just before the drug is due will provide the lowest or 'trough' level when the patient is most at risk and the control most vulnerable. Blood should also be taken at 'peak' times, usually 2–3 hours after the dose. Toxic effects are often related to extreme peaks which might be missed if blood sampling is random. Occasionally an arrhythmia 'breaks through' despite treatment. Blood levels at these times are useful to see if therapeutic levels have been achieved. This will help to establish whether the drug has been given in an inadequate dosage or whether it has failed and another should be selected.

Coronary Care Unit Manual

It is recommended that all coronary care units have a policy and therapeutic manual for the instruction and guidance of its staff. This should not attempt to cover all aspects in depth, but should provide a working basis for the frequently changing junior medical and nursing staff. Each patient is an individual and may present problems particular to his own circumstances. A manual should therefore indicate guidelines and not a set of rules. The following drug information has been abstracted from the current manual in use on the coronary care unit at the Regional Cardiothoracic Centre, Freeman Hospital, Newcastle upon Tyne.

INDIVIDUAL DRUGS — PRESCRIBING AND CLINICAL INFORMATION

Amiodarone

This drug has Class III action, but it may have Class I properties when given intravenously. It is slow to achieve therapeutic effect when given orally which limits its oral use in acute situations. It is effective against a wide range of arrhythmias involving atria, ventricles and accessory pathways. However, it is better reserved for those refractory to other treatment because of relatively high incidence of side-effects.

Dosage   : IV Loading requires a total of 1.5 g given over 24 hours. This commences with 7 mg/kg by infusion over 30 minutes, the remainder of the total loading dose being given over the next 23 hours.
                          : Oral Loading, optimal dose has not yet been established. Varies between 600–1200 mg/day for 3–4 days.
                          : Maintenance therapy 200–600 mg/day orally.
Side-effects   : Hypotension with intravenous infusion, corneal deposits, blue discolouration of skin, photosensitivity, thyroid disorders, pulmonary alveolitis.

Aprindine

This drug has Class I action. It is more useful for ventricular than atrial arrhythmias. It is almost completely absorbed orally and it is metabolised in liver. Its half-life varies from 12–60 hours.

Dosage   : Oral loading dose 200–400 mg
                          : Oral maintenance dose 50–100 mg given twice daily.
Side-effects   : Tremor, dizziness, hallucinations, diplopia, memory impairment, convulsions, nausea, diarrhoea, jaundice, agranulocytosis.

Atropine

This is a parasympathetic blocking drug which is used to increase heart rate when there is symptomatic bradycardia. When sinus bradycardia complicates acute infarction, too large a dose of atropine may result in tachycardia and arrhythmia. It is metabolised in liver.

Dosage   : 0·3–0·6 mg IV. Repeat 0·3 mg IV — every 5 minutes until desired effect or side effects. A maximum total dose of 0·04 mg/kg will achieve total vagal blockade.
Side-effects   : Dry mouth, blurred vision, urinary retention, confusion, hallucinations.

Beta-blocking drugs

These drugs have Class II action. They are used particularly for supraventricular arrhythmias. Poor haemodynamic states often limit their use. Many preparations are available. The following are commonly used:

Dosage

: Practolol — 5 mg IV given over 1–2 minutes. May be repeated every 5 minutes until desired effect or side-effects. Maximum total dose 20 mg.

: Metoprolol — 5 mg IV given over 1–2 minutes. May be repeated every 5 minutes until desired effect or side-effects. Maximum total dose 15 mg.

: Acebutolol — 25 mg IV given over 3–5 minutes. May be repeated using 25 mg by IV infusion over about 1 hour. Maximum total dose 100 mg.

: Atenolol — 2·5 mg IV given over 2–3 minutes. May be repeated every 5 minutes until desired effect or side-effects. Maximum total dose 10 mg.

Side-effects

: Hypotension, bradycardia after reversion of arrhythmia, bronchospasm.

Bretylium

This drug has Class II and III actions. It inhibits release of noradrenaline from nerve endings and blocks noradrenaline uptake. It is sometimes effective in suppressing recurrent ventricular arrhythmias. There is incomplete oral absorption so parenteral administration is required. It is excreted unchanged in urine. Its half-life when given IM is 4–16 hours (mean 10 hours).

Dosage

: If urgent, 5–10 mg/kg given IV over 1 minute.

: If less urgent, 5–10 mg/kg may be given by IV infusion over 10 minutes. This may be repeated every 15–30 minutes to maximum total dose of 30 mg/kg.

: To maintain effect, 5–10 mg/kg IV or

IM every 6–8 hours. Total 24 hour dose
should not exceed 30 mg/kg.

Side-effects
: Hypotension due to adrenergic blockade. With IV bolus, nausea and vomiting, transient increase in blood pressure
due to release of noradrenaline.

Digoxin

This drug possesses three important properties affecting supraventricular tissue, namely shortening atrial refractoriness,
speeding atrial conduction and slowing AV conduction. These
properties are important in either stopping atrial arrhythmias or
slowing the ventricular rate. In acute infarction, these arrhythmias may be due to left ventricular failure and atrial distension.
The positive inotropic effect of digoxin improves left ventricular
function and reduces atrial stretch, thus reducing the likelihood of
supraventricular arrhythmias.

Its onset of action is 30 min when given by mouth, 15 min when
given IV. Its peak action is at 6 hours when given by mouth, 2
hours IV. Its half-life is about 33 hours with normal renal function. Body weight determines the loading dose and renal function
influences maintenance dose.

Dosage
: Loading dose IV, 0·5 mg by infusion
over 30 minutes. Repeat infusion of
0·25–0·5 mg 6–8 hours later. Usual total
IV dose required in first 24 hours is
0·5–1·5 mg.
: Loading dose orally, 0·5–1·0 mg in 24
hours.
: Maintenance 0·125–0·375 mg/day orally.

Side-effects
: Anorexia, nausea, vomiting, diarrhoea.
Extra-systoles and ectopic tachycardia,
particularly paroxysmal atrial tachycardia with block. Conduction defects,
mostly involving the AV node.

Disopyramide

Disopyramide has Class I action with additional vagal inhibiting
effect. Its main function is for ventricular arrhythmias, although it

is useful but less effective with atrial arrhythmias. It is 50% excreted in the urine and 50% metabolised in the liver. Its half-life is 6 hours, but this may be increased in infarction. Well-absorbed, its peak blood levels occur within 2 hours.

Dosage : Loading dose 0·5 mg/kg IV over 5 minutes. Continue with 1·0 mg/kg/hour IV for 3 hours.

: Maintenance therapy may be given IV 0·4 mg/kg/hour or orally 300–800 mg/ 24 hours at 6–8 hour intervals.

Side-effects : Hypotension, heart failure, widening of QRS complexes, atropine-like effects, bradycardia if sinus node disease.

Encainide

Class I action. New drug effective chiefly in ventricular arrhythmias. Infrequently, the arrhythmia may be aggravated.

Dosage : Loading 0·25 mg IV or orally. Repeat in 6 hours.

: Maintenance — 100–300 mg/day given 4–6 hourly.

Side-effects : QRS widening, worsening of arrhythmia, headache, nausea dizziness.

Flecainide

Class I action. New drug effective chiefly in ventricular arrhythmias. Significantly slows retrograde conduction at the AV junction making it valuable in re-entry arrhythmias at this site.

Dosage : The following IV regime achieves a therapeutic effect over 3 hours; 30 mg bolus followed by 12 mg infusion over first hour, then a further 30 mg bolus followed by 24 mg infusion over second hour, then a final 30 mg bolus followed by 36 mg infusion over third hour.

: Oral maintenance 100–200 mg given twice daily.

Side-effects : Dizziness, blurred vision, headache, disorientation, drowsiness, nausea, paraesthesia, negative inotropc effects.

Lignocaine

Lignocaine has Class I action. It is the drug of choice for ventricular arrhythmias complicating acute myocardial infarction. It has a rapid onset of action when given IV which lasts only 15–20 min. It requires a maintenance infusion to sustain effect. It is metabolised in liver. It causes no significant depression of LV function.

Dosage
: To terminate an arrhythmia — 50 mg IV given over 1 minute. Repeat after 2 minutes. If required, repeat 25 mg IV every 2 minutes up to a total of 2·0–2·5 mg/kg (approximately 150–175 mg).
: To prevent an arrhythmia — 50 mg IV over 1 minute and repeat after 2 minutes.
: In either of the above situations, IV maintenance can be achieved with the infusion of 4 mg/min for 30 minutes. Then 3 mg/min for 30 minutes and
: 2 mg/min thereafter.
: Early recurrence of arrhythmias — 25–30 mg IV and maintain same infusion rate.
: Late recurrence of arrhythmia — 25–30 mg IV and increase infusion rate.
: Reduced requirements in heart failure, chronic liver disease.

Side-effects
: Nausea, vomiting, numbness, tingling and glossal paraesthesia. CNS excitation or depression, particularly in elderly.

Mexiletine

Mexiletine has Class I action and is effective against ventricular arrhythmias. It may be effective given IV when lignocaine has failed. It is metabolised in the liver.

Dosage
: IV loading dose, 8 mg/min for 30 minutes, the 1·5 mg/min for 2 hours, then 1·0 mg/min for 8 hours.
: IV maintenance 0·5–1·0 mg/min by infusion.

	: Oral loading with 400–600 mg initial dose followed by 200 mg 2 hours and 4 hours later.
	: Oral maintenance 200–250 mg given 8 hourly.
Side-effects	: Nausea, vomiting, tremor, nystagmus, dizziness, drowsiness, blurred vision, hypotension, bradycardia.

Phenytoin

This drug has Class I action. It is a last-line drug for ventricular arrhythmias and is ineffective for atrial arrhythmias. It is useful for digoxin-toxic ventricular arrhythmias. It has variable small bowel absorption and is metabolised in the liver.

Dosage	: 100 mg IV every 5 minutes until reversion of arrhythmia or side-effects, up to a total of 1 g.
	: Oral loading regime, 1 g first day, 500 mg second day and third day given in divided doses 6 hourly.
	: Oral maintenance 300–400 mg/day in divided doses.
Side-effects	: Respiratory arrest and bradycardia with IV therapy. Hypotension, drowsiness, nystagmus, vertigo.

Procainamide

This drug has Class I action and is useful for atrial and ventricular arrhythmias. It is well-absorbed with peak levels occurring in 1 hour. It is metabolised at variable rates in the liver, toxic effects being more common when liver metabolism is slow. The metabolite is active and is excreted through kidney. Excretion is delayed with cardio-renal impairment and alkaline urine. Blood levels of the drug should be taken (toxic > 12 mg/litre).

Dosage	: 100 mg IV every 5 minutes up to maximum of 1 g, until reversion of arrhythmia or hypotension or QRS widening occurs.
	: IV maintenance 1·5–5·0 mg/min by infusion.
	: Oral loading dose 2 g in Durule form.

Oral maintenance 1·5 g Durules 8 hourly.

Side-effects : Anorexia, nausea, vomiting, hypotension, QRS widening, asystole. Allergic reactions (fever and rashes). Lupus syndrome.

Quinidine

Quinidine has Class I action. It is valuable for atrial and ventricular arrhythmias. Its anticholinergic effect improves AV node conduction and may increase heart rate. It is metabolised in liver. Quinidine has rapid and complete absorption with peak levels in 1–2 hours. Its half-life is 4–6 hours. Quinidine bisulphate is a long-acting sustained release preparation.

Dosage : Oral loading dose with quinidine sulphate 200 mg 2 hourly up to total of 5 doses or until side-effects appear.

: Oral loading dose with quinidine bisulphate 750–1000 mg.

: Oral maintenance with quinidine bisulphate 1·0–2·5 g/day given at 12 hourly divided doses.

Side-effects : Anorexia, nausea, vomiting, diarrhoea. Allergic reactions (fever, urticaria, rashes). Immunological abnormalities (marrow depression). QT prolongation, ventricular arrhythmias and syncope.

Tocainide

This drug has Class I action. It is effective against ventricular arrhythmias and is useful when they are refractory to other drugs. It is well-absorbed with peak levels in 60–90 min. It is 60% metabolised by the liver and 40% excreted by the kidneys. Its half-life is 10–17 hours.

Dosage : Oral loading dose 400–800 mg.

: IV loading dose 0·5–0·75 mg/kg/min for 15 min.

: Oral maintenance dose 400–600 mg 8 hourly.

Side-effects : Drowsiness, paraesthesia, tremor, incoordination, anorexia, vomiting, constipation, allergy (maculopapular rash).

Verapamil

Verapamil has Class 4 action. It is a calcium antagonist with its main effect on arrhythmias involving the AV node, particularly the re-entrant type. It is dangerous in patients on oral beta-blockers or who have been given IV beta-blockers as it may produce extreme bradycardia and hypotension. It has rapid absorption.

Dosage   : 5–10 mg IV over 5 minutes to terminate arrhythmia. May be repeated after 30 minutes.
                      : Oral maintenance 40–160 mg 8 hourly.
Side-effects   : Nausea, constipation, headache, dizziness, skin rashes.

MANAGEMENT OF SPECIFIC ARRHYTHMIAS

Sinus Bradycardia

Sinus bradycardia is defined as sinus rhythm with a persistent rate of less than 60 beats/min. Treatment is required if:

1. symptomatic — light headed, particularly when bradycardia is marked or there are sinus pauses.
2. hypotension.
3. associated with ventricular extrasystoles, which may progress to more serious ventricular arrhythmias.

Treatment for sinus bradycardia is:

1. atropine.
2. isoprenaline infusion.
3. temporary cardiac pacing.

Sinus Tachycardia

Sinus tachycardia is defined as sinus rhythm with a persistent rate greater than 100 beats/min. It is invariably due to increased sympathetic stimulation following a large myocardial infarction.

It may also be due to anxiety, pain or complication of infarction, such as mitral regurgitation or pericarditis. Occasionally, the degree of tachycardia appears inappropriate to the patient's otherwise satisfactory state and beta-blocking agents can be used cautiously to reduce the rate. This would particularly be considered if ventricular extrasystoles were present. Sinus tachycardia should always prompt a careful search for an underlying cause.
Treatment:

1. Pain relief when appropriate.
2. Reassurance and sedation when appropriate.
3. Treatment of identified cause.
4. Consider use of beta-blockers.

Supraventricular Extrasystoles

Supraventricular extrasystoles rarely require treatment and can usually be ignored. If frequency increases, it may indicate possible development of atrial fibrillation. Digoxin, disopyramide, quinidine and amiodarone would be effective.

Atrial Fibrillation

This is usually due to left ventricular failure, pericarditis or atrial infarction. Management is determined by the haemodynamic state of the patient, the heart rate and whether the rhythm is sustained or paroxysmal.
Treatment:

1. Satisfactory clinical state with rate less than 100 beats/min — No treatment necessary.
2. Satisfactory clinical state with rate greater than 100 beats/min:
   - Digoxin
   - Verapamil
   - Disopyramide
   - Beta-blocking agent, possibly with digoxin.
3. Deteriorating haemodynamic state — cardioversion.
4. Consider prophylactic use of anticoagulants.

Atrial Flutter

The management of atrial flutter is similar to atrial fibrillation.

The heart rate may be more difficult to control with digoxin. Cardioversion may be considered earlier. Atrial pacing may either revert the flutter to sinus rhythm or to atrial fibrillation which is easier to control. Amiodarone is effective in preventing recurrent atrial flutter.

Supraventricular Tachycardia

This is usually associated with a fast heart rate and requires treatment:

1. Carotid sinus massage.
2. IV verapamil — probably the first choice of drug.
3. Digoxin and beta-blocking drugs will slow AV conduction and reduce heart rate.
4. IV disopyramide and procainamide are likely to restore sinus rhythm.
5. Cardioversion or atrial pacing.

Ventricular Extrasystoles

The first important question to be answered about ventricular extrasystoles is whether or not they require treatment. The concept that ventricular extrasystoles were a warning of the possible development of more serious arrhythmias was the basis of early aggressive treatment to suppress them. This has recently been questioned and will be discussed in more detail in Chapter 16. Short runs, R on T type and more than 5 per minute have conventionally been regarded as indications for treatment.

1. Lignocaine, loading dose plus infusion.
2. Second line drugs (see Ventricular Tachycardia).

Ventricular Tachycardia

This is defined as three or more consecutive ventricular extrasystoles at a rate of 120 per minute or greater. It may not require treatment if it is short, isolated and asymptomatic. However, recurrent episodes may lead to VF and need suppression. Serum potassium and magnesium levels should be checked in ventricular tachycardia.

Reversion — 1. Lignocaine
2. Cardioversion if the haemodynamic state is poor.

Second line drugs — 1. Procainamide
2. Disopyramide
3. Mexiletine
4. Flecainide
5. Amiodarone
6. Bretylium
7. Phenytoin

Cardiac pacing using overdrive suppression can sometimes be helpful in reverting an episode of ventricular tachycardia.

Prophylaxis — If the arrhythmia occurs early (< 24 hours) after infarction, long-term treatment may not be required. If it is a later complication, lignocaine should be followed by one of the second line drugs noted above. Repetitive late ventricular tachycardia may be difficult to prevent and control and may require specialised haemodynamic and electrophysiological investigation.

Ventricular Fibrillation

This has been discussed in detail in Chapter 6.

OTHER IMPORTANT DRUGS COMMONLY USED IN THE CCU

Adrenaline

This drug may be required during cardiac arrest, either to provoke some electrical activity in the case of asystole or to coarsen ventricular fibrillation if cardioversion is initially unsuccessful. It may be given IV or by intracardiac injection.

Dosage   : 10 ml of 1:10 000 solution.

Diamorphine

This is the most widely used analgesic for relief of pain of infarction. It is valuable also in patients distressed by left ventricular failure and nocturnal dyspnoea. It is commonly diluted with 12·5 mg prochlorperazine to prevent nausea and vomiting.

Dosage	: 5 mg IV over 2–3 min. May be repeated in doses of 2·5 mg every 10–15 min up to 15 mg or until adequate pain relief is achieved.
Side-effects	: Nausea, vomiting, respiratory depression, delayed gastric emptying, coma.
Antagonist	: Naloxone, usually 0·4–1·2 mg.

Dopamine

This is a naturally occurring catecholamine found in sympathetic nerves and adrenal glands. Its actions depend upon the infusion rate. At slow rates (< 4 µg/kg/min), dopamine dilates renal and systemic vessels and is helpful in resistant heart failure. Faster rates of infusion (4–10 µg/kg/min) increase cardiac output, contractility and heart rate. Still higher rates may cause vasoconstriction and reduce renal blood flow.

| Dosage | : Dilute in 5% dextrose and give through a central line at 1–2 µg/kg/min. Increase every 15–30 min by 1–4 µg/kg/min up to 50 µg/kg/min. |
| Side-effects | : Sinus tachycardia, arrhythmias. Local extravasation may cause tissue necrosis and can be reversed by infiltration with phentolamine. There may be rebound hypotension on withdrawal so dopamine should be discontinued gradually. |

Dobutamine

This drug is similar to dopamine, but is a direct-acting agent and does not cause release of endogenous noradrenaline. It has less sinus tachycardia and arrhythmia potential. It is preferred by some physicians for the low output and heart failure associated with myocardial infarction.

| Dosage | : 2·5–10 µg/kg/min, given diluted intravenously. |
| Side-effects | : Nausea, headache, angina, palpitations, dyspnoea. |

Heparin

The following factors predispose to venous thrombosis: advanced age, obesity, pre-existing venous disease, previous venous thrombosis, slowness to mobilise, cardiac failure or shock. Systemic embolism is liable to occur with atrial fibrillation and aneurysm.

Low-dose heparin prophylaxis	: 10 000–15 000 units/day given by SC injections every 8–12 hours.
Full-dose heparin	: Either intermittent IV injections or continuous infusion: 5 000 units IV every 4 hours. Bolus 5 000 units with maintenance infusion of 30 000 units in 24 hours. The dose may be changed according to blood tests, so frequently checking with haematology laboratory is necessary.
Side-effects	: Haemorrhage, thrombocytopenia.

Isoprenaline

This is most commonly required for treatment of bradycardia or asystole while setting up for a temporary pacemaker.

Dosage	: Initial bolus of 0·1 mg IV. Then give infusion of 2 mg in 500 ml 5% dextrose (= 4 µg/ml) set at initial rate of 1 µg/min. Increase as necessary to 20 µg/min or until sinus tachycardia or arrhythmias appear.
Note	: Larger doses are required if the patient is receiving beta-blockers.
Side-effects	: Palpitations, sinus tachycardia, arrhythmias.

Isosorbide

Isosorbide is a vasodilator with its primary effect on veins and to a lesser extent on arteries. It may be used by IV infusion to treat unresponsive heart failure and acute coronary insufficiency.

Dosage	: Infusion commencing at 10 µg/min. Increase by 10 µg/min until desired effect or side-effects appear.
Side-effects	: Headache, hypotension, sinus tachycardia.

Labetalol

This drug blocks both alpha and beta sympathetic receptors. It is useful to control hypertension following myocardial infarction and to lower blood pressure in dissecting aneurysm.

Dosage
: Infusion commencing at 1 mg/min. Increase by 1 mg/min every 30 min until desired effect appears or up to a maximum of 5 mg/min.

Side-effects
: Nausea, vomiting, epigastric discomfort, scalp tingling.

Salbutamol

This drug reduces systemic arterial resistance and is useful in patients with low cardiac output and heart failure after infarction.

Dosage
: 5 µg/min increasing to maximum of 50 µg/min, diluted in 5% dextrose. Its effects should be followed by haemodynamic monitoring.

Side-effects
: Sinus tachycardia, arrhythmias, hypotension.

Sodium Nitroprusside

This is a powerful vasodilator mainly used to control hypertensive emergencies. It has a rapid onset of action. It reduces the pressure against which the heart has to pump and thus is useful in the management of heart failure. It should be diluted in 5% dextrose and wrapped in foil to protect it from light. It must be used within 4 hours of preparation.

Dosage
: 0·5–1·5 µg/min by IV infusion, controlled by haemodynamic monitoring.

Side-effects
: Hypotension. It is converted to cyanide by red blood cells and prolonged use may lead to poisoning, the symptoms of which are tachycardia, dizziness, sweating, hypoventilation, acidosis, coma.

16

Modern Trends in Coronary Artery Disease

Echocardiography

The technique of examining the heart's structure and function using sound waves has been gradually gaining momentum since its introduction in the mid-1950s. This facility allows non-invasive and repeated evaluation at minimal patient inconvenience, which is particularly welcome in an acute coronary care setting. Echocardiography has developed from sound radar (sonar) used in wartime to detect submarines and commercially in the fishing industry. A hand-held transducer which emits ultrasound pulses is applied to the chest over the heart. When this wave of energy meets tissue in the heart with differing acoustic properties, some will be reflected back towards the transducer and can be recorded on an oscilloscope. A series of 'spikes' will be seen which represent the echoes returning from different levels of the heart — this is called the A-mode display. Since the structures within the heart are constantly moving, the position of the spikes will vary and this can be better appreciated on the M-mode or motion display. This can be recorded on light sensitive paper to provide a permanent record. By aiming the transducer at different parts of the heart, the position and movement of the various cardiac structures can be studied.

More recently, electronic developments have enabled the ultrasound beam to scan rapidly across the heart and produce two dimensional (2–D) images. The heart can be seen to contract and relax as clearly as on angiograms and normal and abnormal movements of valves can be identified.

There is no doubt that echocardiography, particularly in the 2–D form, has been a major advance in cardiology and has obviated the need for cardiac catheterisation in many patients. On the CCU it can provide valuable information about cardiac function in the acutely ill patient. After infarction, abnormalities of regional wall movement of the left ventricle can be detected and the extent of damage evaluated. Pericardial effusions can be easily seen and occasionally abnormalities of the aortic root are evident as in the case of dissecting aneurysms. Echocardiography may also clarify the cause of systolic murmurs developing during infarction, since acquired VSDs and mitral regurgitation due to papillary muscle rupture may show characteristic abnormalities. At present the technique is unable to provide any direct evidence of coronary artery disease, although left main stem stenosis has occasionally been seen. A full evaluation of the extent of coronary artery involvement still requires cardiac catheterisation and coronary angiography.

Nuclear Medicine and Coronary Artery Disease

The development of radiopharmaceutics and nuclear medicine instrumentation over the last 10 to 15 years has provided an important non-invasive technique to study cardiac function. If a radioactive tracer is given by intravenous injection, it will be distributed throughout the body and can be detected by scanning techniques. Those organs with a large blood flow will receive a proportionally large amount of the tracer which will be evenly distributed within them. If there were a regional abnormality of blood flow within an organ, as would occur in the myocardium with ischaemia or infarction, the isotope would not accumulate in these areas and 'cold spots' would appear.

Thallium-201 is most commonly used for detecting abnormalities of myocardial perfusion. An exercise stress test is performed in the usual way and thallium is given intravenously at peak exercise or development of angina. The patient continues to exercise for a further minute and then stops. He is then positioned on a trolley under a scintillation camera which picks up the emission from the isotope. With computer enhancement, this is displayed on a screen and shows the areas of normal perfusion.

Cold spots of poor uptake can be identified and characteristic patterns can be related to individual coronary artery lesions. Scans repeated several hours later may also be helpful. If a defect persists, it will be due to infarction, whereas when ischaemia resolves, redistribution will take place and the initial defect will disappear.

Radioisotopes have also proved helpful in diagnosing acute myocardial infarction when ECG and enzyme changes are equivocal. Some isotopes, for example technesium-labelled pyrophosphate, concentrate in acutely damaged tissue and would appear as a hot spot in an area of myocardial infarction. This would be shown in almost all transmural infarctions and the majority of subendocardial infarctions 24–48 hours after the onset of pain. A totally normal scan would suggest a less than 5% chance of infarction.

When a tracer has become equally distributed in the blood (equilibration), it can provide information about ventricular function. This is referred to as a blood pool scan. Repeated images triggered from the ECG are rapidly recorded from the heart and can be displayed on a cine film. This allows evaluation of ventricular size, function and regional wall movement. Technesium-labelled albumin is commonly used and the technique is known as a MUGA (multiple gated acquisition) SCAN.

Radioactive tracer techniques have become established in the evaluation of cardiac function and structure. The size of the equipment has become smaller and now portable units are available for use on coronary care units, allowing repeated investigations and avoiding invasive techniques.

Coronary Angioplasty

Angioplasty is the term given to the technique of compressing an area of atheroma in an artery to reduce the obstruction to blood flow. Only in the later 1970s was it developed for use in the coronary arteries, however, it has been widely adopted throughout the world in a relatively short time. A coronary angiogram catheter, slightly larger than usual, is passed from the femoral or brachial artery and advanced to the ostium of the appropriate coronary artery. This serves as a guide for a smaller dilating catheter which is passed up within it. The dilating catheter has an inflatable balloon close to its tip and when the dilating catheter has been advanced into the coronary branch and through the stenosis, the balloon is inflated to compress and flatten the narrowing.

At first this technique was reserved for patients with a short history of angina, good left ventricular function and single vessel non-calcified disease. As experience was gained and the success rate increased, the indications for the procedure were widened and the technique was used in patients with more severe disease. Now, it is common for more than one stenosis to be dilated during the procedure and areas of narrowing within coronary artery grafts can also be relieved.

However, the technique is not without risks. It should only be undertaken in centres regularly performing cardiac catheterisation and coronary angiography and the immediate availability of a cardiac surgical team is essential. Attempts to dilate stenoses may damage the coronary artery which may then become obstructed. Without urgent surgery and bypass grafting, a large infarction could occur. The incidence of major complications producing severe ischaemia, myocardial infarction or death is probably comparable to that of coronary artery surgery. Successful angioplasty relieves angina as effectively as surgery with the obvious advantages of avoiding an open heart operation. If symptoms recur, a repeat dilatation may be possible.

It is likely that as experience is more widely gained and the equipment and technique refined, many more patients will be regarded as suitable for angioplasty, who at present wait for surgery. In addition some patients, who might be regarded as at high risk or unsuitable for surgery because of other medical conditions, could benefit from this procedure.

Current Use of Aspirin

The role of antiplatelet agents in the secondary prevention of myocardial infarction and sudden death has been extensively studied with disappointing results. While some benefit has been noted using aspirin and dipyridamole, the results in the past have not been of statistical significance. The doses used were high (900–1500 mg/day) and side-effects were observed. It should be noted that any benefit has been confined to men.

A recent study using a lower dose of buffered aspirin (324 mg/day) reported a reduction of 50% in the incidence of infarction and sudden death in men with unstable angina, if the drug was prescribed soon after admission and continued for 12 days. This appears promising for patients with unstable angina.

The use of antiplatelet therapy in the primary prevention of myocardial infarction has received less study and results are not significant.

Intracoronary Thrombolysis

In most patients who sustain a myocardial infarction, a fresh thrombus at the site of previous atheromatous narrowing appears to be responsible. Although the concept of dissolving clot (lysis) had been applied at other sites, only recently has the value of this been explored in the coronary arteries. There is now no doubt that in the majority of patients, streptokinase infused into the obstructed coronary vessel will restore blood flow. After the initial enthusiasm, however, it became clear that there were important questions to answer before it became widely adopted. The risk of coronary angiography during the early phase of an evolving infarction was not as high as might have been anticipated, but evidence of benefit was required to justify the procedure. Clearly the longer the time elapsed before restoration of blood flow, the less likely was the procedure to result in improved myocardial function. Most workers have regarded it as desirable to achieve lysis within 3 hours of the onset of symptoms, which poses obvious problems in organisation.

Nevertheless, studies have been completed to suggested that early intervention is feasible, relatively safe and of potential benefit. In some cases, restoring blood flow has been associated with relief of pain and reduction of ST elevation. Radioisotope studies have shown improved coronary blood flow and regional wall movement suggesting maintained functional benefit. However, there is a definite mortality and morbidity associated with the procedure, probably greater than would have been anticipated from the infarction alone.

At present, intracoronary thrombolysis is restricted in its application to those patients who present early during infarction to specialised centres with immediate availability of their facilities. Under these circumstances, it is unlikely to offer a realistic solution. However, if a safe and effective thrombolytic preparation becomes available which can be given intravenously, it would potentially increase the number of patients who might benefit from this approach.

Reducing the Size of an Infarction

This is an area which is exciting much research and controversy. Since mortality is related to infarct size, the concept of giving a drug in the early stages of a myocardial infarction to limit the size of the ultimate area of damage is attractive. Although there are important differences, a similar concept evolved to protect the arrested heart during open heart surgery. Previously, simple cardiac arrest during cardiopulmonary bypass only allowed about one hour before major ischaemic injury developed, whereas the use of a cold protective solution (cardioplegia) at the onset of arrest, has extended this to several hours.

Much of the early experimental work in animals in the early 1970s was encouraging and many agents were identified which appeared to have a beneficial effect. However, none have been introduced into regular clinical practice as yet. Some now question whether it is possible to achieve this goal and suggest that agents which delay the harmful effects of ischaemia are of no value when the arterial supply is obstructed and infarction is inevitable. Even with cold cardioplegia during open heart surgery, damage would eventually occur if the coronary blood flow were not normally restored.

It is conceivable that, in the more specialised cardiac centres, a combined approach of giving a drug to delay damage and then attempting to restore regional blood flow by streptokinase, angio-plasty or coronary artery bypass grafting, might limit the size of an evolving infarction. However, this could only be applied to a small number of patients. The time has not yet arrived when a drug can be given to all patients suspected of having an infarction, wherever they may be, with a proven realistic change of reducing the area of necrosis.

Warning Arrhythmias in Acute Myocardial Infarction

Since the early years of coronary care units, it has been appreciated that ventricular extrasystoles and ventricular fibrillation are common during acute infarction. As the first ECG complex of fibrillation is indeed an extrasystole, it was postulated that extrasystoles should be treated to prevent fibrillation developing. Monitoring the patients' ECGs on the oscilloscope suggested that certain types of extrasystoles were particularly dangerous (Lown *et al.*, 1967) and it became routine to give lignocaine when five or more were seen in a minute, when they fell on the T wave of the preceding sinus beat, or when they were multifocal or occurred in runs. The incidence of ventricular fibrillation was reduced and was presumed to be due to this effective management.

A number of observations later suggested that it was not quite this simple. Some patients appeared to develop ventricular fibrillation without any warning extrasystoles and occasionally fibrillation was initiated by extrasystoles falling well after the T wave. Indeed, it was suggested that the warning arrhythmias used for so long as the basis of CCU management were as frequent in patients who did not go on to develop fibrillation and were not, therefore, a good predictive guide (Lie *et al.*, 1975; El Sherif *et al.*, 1976). More recently, it has been shown retrospectively that R on T extrasystoles occur more frequently during the 10 minutes before fibrillation develops, but that this would be difficult to recognise and probably would not give enough time for treatment to be started (Campbell, 1981). These studies have relied on different recording techniques to reach their conclusions. It has been appreciated that visual monitoring of the oscilloscope is unreliable and many events will be missed. Continuous tape recording of ECGs and computer analysis has permitted a much more detailed and accurate evaluation of so called 'warning arrhythmias' and has shown that at present there is no useful way of reliably predicting which patient will develop primary ventricular fibrillation.

Many CCUs have, therefore, changed their strategy. Some have joined the search for a drug which can safely be given to all patients and others have preferred to ignore all asymptomatic ventricular arrhythmias. Unfortunately, no drug has yet been shown to reduce ventricular fibrillation, which would be suitable and free from side-effects for all patients both in and out of hospital. Since many patients die before they reach hospital, a simple regime suitable for delivery at home or in an ambulance would be required if it were to have any useful impact. Also it would be essential for the drug not to have any significant myocardial depressant effect in those patients with large infarctions who border on heart failure. Finally, if a cover-all prophylactic policy is adopted, the drug will inevitably be given to many patients who ultimately are shown not to have sustained in infarction. So far, only lignocaine given IV in high dosage has been shown in a controlled study to convincingly reduce ventricular fibrillation in hospital (Lie *et al.*, 1974; Wyman *et al.*, 1974). Although reported side-effects were common with high dosage, the encouraging response was not found when the drug was given intramuscularly (Lie *et al.*, 1978). Many other potentially valuable drugs, suitable for use outside hospital, have been studied. While they have reduced ventricular arrhythmias, they have not statistically affected the incidence of ventricular fibrillation. The studies quoted, employing continuous ECG tape recordings, have not only denied the concept of warning arrhythmias, but also clarified the incidence of ventricular arrhythmias during the first 24 hours after infarction. Single or paired ventricular extrasystoles occur in almost all patients and three or more consecutive extrasystoles (VT) in about 75%. Longer paroxysms of VT (10 or more complexes) are seen in about 25%. Reports of ventricular fibrillation vary between 5–10%. There is a danger, therefore, of reacting inappropriately to some ventricular arrhythmias which are common and innocent. Since it has been shown that patients who have been promptly and effectively resuscitated from primary ventricular fibrillation progress as well as other infarct patients, it is very reasonable to await this arrhythmia and defibrillate it. Then clearly, only patients who require treatment receive it and others avoid unnecessary therapy. It is, however, only appropriate to adopt this policy in a coronary care unit setting with staff confident in their ability to act effectively at any time throughout a 24 hour period.

Implanted Defibrillator

The concept of patients who are prone to recurrent ventricular fibrillation, carrying an automatic defibrillating device capable of restoring sinus rhythm, is now reality. Electronic miniaturisation has permitted the development of a defibrillator about the size of a pacemaker. This is implanted beneath the skin and is connected to a mesh electrode which is stitched onto the heart. Circuits in the unit constantly monitor cardiac electrical activity and can detect ventricular fibrillation. It then delivers a shock and invariably reverts the arrhythmia. Following early experimental work with animals, it has now been applied in the clinical situation in high risk patients with encouraging results. Further clinical evaluation is in progress.

Surgery for Arrhythmias

Generally, drug treatment is the preferred method of dealing with cardiac arrhythmias. Some forms of tachycardia may however be extremely difficult to control by conventional means and may be responsible for much distress, sometimes due to side-effects of the drugs used. It is important to appreciate that surgery has gradually evolved to offer a very real alternative to some patients with resistant life-threatening arrhythmias. The operations rely on two basic principles. First, to remove tissue which initiates the arrhythmia by enhanced automaticity and second, to interrupt pathways used to sustain the arrhythmia by the re-entry mechanism.

Surgical division of the accessory pathway in the WPW syndrome removes one of the limbs of the re-entry pathway and will prevent a very rapid ventricular response to atrial fibrillation. This can now be achieved with a high success rate and relative safety. Problems due to resistant supraventricular tachycardia in patients without pre-excitation can be managed by ablation of the AV node to produce complete heart block. The tachycardia will then be unable to conduct to the ventricles. However, it will be necessary to implant a permanent pacemaker to maintain a satisfactory heart rate.

Resistant ventricular arrhythmias are most commonly related to coronary artery disease, often occurring as a late problem after myocardial infarction. They are sometimes a feature of aneurysm formation and may be cured by its resection. It is now appreciated that the areas responsible for the arrhythmia may lie along the margins of the aneurysm and the problem may not be solved unless these areas also are removed. Arrhythmia surgery will require specialised electrophysiological mapping procedures to determine the site of origin of the tachycardia and the way it spreads through the ventricles. With this information, the surgeon can remove the areas responsible or make an incision (ventriculotomy) to prevent a re-entry arrhythmia. Sometimes quite large areas of the endocardium have to be resected for the procedure to be successful and the ventriculotomy may need to encircle the ventricle to isolate the ectopic focus. These arrhythmias are not confined to patients with advanced heart disease and may occasionally be found in patients with little or no other abnormality.

At present these techniques are employed by only a few special-ised cardiac centres. Nevertheless, it is important to appreciate that they are available and offer an alternative method of manage-ment for some difficult arrhythmia problems.

Selecting Patients for Coronary Artery Surgery

The primary aim of coronary artery bypass grafting is the relief of angina. The failure of medical treatment to improve angina and restore the patient to an acceptable level of activity is the main indication to consider a surgical solution. Since patients' persona-lities, ages, occupations and recreational activities vary consider-ably, the definition of 'failed medical treatment' will vary from patient to patient. What is an acceptable level of restriction for one individual may be totally unacceptable to another.

Another important consideration is whether successful surgery improves prognosis when compared with medical treatment. It has now been established that this is indeed the situation for two well-defined groups: first, those patients with significant left main stem stenosis and second, those with significant stenoses affecting all three major coronary artery branches (triple vessel disease).

Therefore, when a patient presents with chest pain, it is impor-tant not only to make a correct diagnosis and institute treatment but also, if ischaemic heart disease is confirmed, to evaluate the extent of the coronary artery involvement. This can only be established with 100% certainty by coronary angiography, but it is impractical to undertake this in every patient with angina.

Exercise stress testing has proved to be a most valuable screen-ing test to separate these patients with severe and extensive disease from those with prognostically less important lesions. In hospital practice, patients with symptomatic coronary artery disease will present in one of two settings. Stable angina is a frequent out-patient problem whereas acute coronary insufficiency and infarc-tion tends to precipitate admissions to CCUs. Exercise testing has a role to play in both situations, but is handled somewhat dif-ferently.

In out-patients a maximal stress test is usually desirable, pro-vided that the necessary precautions are taken. Those patients who demonstrate a strongly positive result with a short exercise time are usually selected for coronary angiography. It would clearly be undesirable and dangerous to subject unstable and infarction patients to such a test. It has become apparent, however, that a limited exercise test can be safely performed as early as one week after an uncomplicated myocardial infarction and may give valuable information about left ventricular function and the extent of coronary artery disease. A positive early test may prompt the doctor to recommend further investigation even though the patient appears to be making satisfactory progress. If the early test is negative, it may be repeated to a higher work load later during convalescence.

As the natural history of coronary artery disease is better defined in relationship to the extent of the disease, further subgroups may be identified which require more aggressive investigation and treatment. Determining which patients fall into higher risk categories and whether their prognosis can be improved by surgery is an important part of their management.

Heart Transplantation

This is a subject that has excited much controversy and objections to it have been made on moral, religious and economic grounds. Considerable publicity accompanied the first human transplant in 1967, but we are now in a better position to evaluate the role it can play in patients with end-stage cardiac disease. With improved methods of detecting and treating rejection, survival has increased and Dr Shumway's unit in Stanford, California has achieved a figure of nearly 40% survival at five years after the operation. When it is considered that patients are not suitable for any other form of treatment, there seems little doubt that the procedure prolongs life. Many have been able to return to work with a substantial reduction or elimination of symptoms.

There are, however, many medical problems. There are many more potential recipients than there are donors and the mortality rate is high. Rejection and intercurrent infection continue to be a problem and the frequent occurrence of coronary artery disease developing in the donor heart after transplantation is now recognised. Hypertension and malignant disease are also seen and are probably related to the treatment given to control rejection.

Most patients who are considered for transplanation are less than 50 years old and have advanced coronary artery disease, usually with repeated infarction and poor left ventricular function or cardiomyopathy with heart failure. The main contraindication is an abnormal pulmonary vasculature with a high pressure or resistance, since the heart is not able to function and heart failure occurs under these circumstances. Many patients have and will benefit from heart transplantation. It is, however, very expensive and time-consuming. If resources are limited, a community and health service will have to consider carefully how to apportion them. Although it is unlikely ever to be cost-effective, the length of survival and improved quality of life now being achieved are impressive.

References

Campbell R.W.F. *et al.* (1981). Ventricular arrhythmias in first twelve hours of acute myocardial infarction: a natural history study. *British Heart Journal;* **46**:351–7.

El-Sherif N. *et al.* (1976). Electrocardiographic antecedents of primary ventricular fibrillation. *British Heart Journal;* **38**:415–22.

Lewis H.D. *et al.* (1983). Protective effects of aspirin against acute myocardial infarction and death in men with unstable angina. *New England Journal of Medicine*; **309**:396–403.

Lie K.I. *et al.* (1974). Lidocaine in the prevention of primary ventricular fibrillation. *New England Journal of Medicine;* **29**:1324–6.

Lie K.I. *et al.* (1975). Observations on patients with primary ventricular fibrillation complicating acute myocardial infarction. *Circulation;* **52**:755–9.

Lie K.I. *et al.* (1978). Efficacy of lidocaine in preventing primary ventricular fibrillation within 1 hour after a 300 mg intramuscular injection. *American Journal of Cardiology;* **41**:674–677.

Lown B. *et al.* (1967). The coronary care unit: new perspectives and directions. *Journal of the American Medical Association;* **199**:188–98.

Wyman M.G. *et al.* (1974). Comprehensive treatment plan for the prevention of primary ventricular fibrillation in acute myocardial infarction. *American Journal of Cardiology*; **33**:661–7.

Index

blood
   flow 9
   tests 60–61
brady-tachy syndrome 159
bretylium 174
British Heart Foundation 124
Bruce protocol 43
bundle of His 10

calcium antagonists 47
cardiac
   arrest 90–93
   arrhythmias 77–94
   cycle 15
   rehabilitation 125
   rupture 71
   vector 27
cardiogenic shock 69–71
cardiomyopathy 161
cardioselective beta blockers 47
care of myocardial infarction
   patient 64–8
carotid sinus massage 84
CCU *see* coronary care unit
Charing Cross IABP 133
chordae tendineae 8
circumflex coronary artery 19
complete heart block 99
conduction
   cells 11
   defects 95–107
congestive cardiomyopathy 161
continuing education 164
contraction cells 11
coronary
   angioplasty 48, 189
   arteriography 44
   artery bypass grafts 48
   care units 1–3
   circulation 18–22
   surgery 196
CPK *see* serum creatinine
   phosphokinase

Datascope IABP system 133

DC conversion 92, 93
defibrillation 92–3
   implanted device 194
demand pacemakers 113
depolarisation 12, 25
diagnosis of angina 40, 44–6
diamorphine 183
diastole 15
diet 65, 127
digoxin 175
disopyramide 175
dissecting aneurysm of the
   aorta 159–160
dobutamine 184–5
dominant coronary artery
   systems 21
dopamine 184
Dressler's syndrome 61, 72
drug classification 168–170
dying heart 89–90

echocardiography 187
Einthoven triangle 28
electrocardiograph
   in angina 41
   in myocardial infarction 52
electrocardiography 23–36
electrode application for ECG 24
electrolyte imbalance 60–61
electrophysiology 12–15, 25
emboli 72–3
encainide 276
endocardium 7
enhanced automaticity 78
erythrocyte sedimentation rate,
   raised 61
ESR *see* erythrocyte sedimentation
   rate
exercise
   effect in angina 39
   programmes 127
   tests 42–3

first degree AV block 96
fixed rate pacemakers 113